Youth Brain Development Correlates

Louies Calderon

Abstract

Adolescence is associated with substantial brain reorganization, and therefore presents a unique period of vulnerability to psychiatric disorders but also a window of opportunity for neuroscience-informed interventions to mitigate the risk of full-blown mental disorders. As such, a comprehensive understanding of adolescent normative brain development and its associated factors are crucial. The doctoral work described herein consists of four studies on the normative trajectories of brain structure and the relation of adolescent brain development to perinatal, physical, psychosocial, cognitive, and environmental factors. First, we used the data from the Enhancing Neuro Imaging Genetics through Meta-Analysis (ENIGMA) lifespan workgroup to construct normative centile curves of brain regions as well as their variation over time, and their inter-individual variability. We then used the IMAGEN longitudinal study of adolescents to characterize the association between developing brain structure and psychopathological traits, neuropsychological measures, and environment using multivariate modeling. We further replicated and expanded on the IMAGEN study by leveraging the phenotypically well-characterized and rich Adolescent Brain Cognitive Development (ABCD) study to investigate the correlates of multimodal brain phenotypes. We hope our findings will

bridge the critical gap in knowledge to advance a biologically informed understanding

of adolescent brain development and will ultimately lend itself to targeted interventions

for improving brain and mental health outcomes.

Table of Contents

Abbreviations

ABCD	Adolescent Brain and Cognitive Development
ACC	Anterior cingulate cortex
AD	Axial diffusivity
ADHD-NF	Attention Deficit Hyperactivity Disorder- Neurofeedback Study
AMC	Amsterdam Medisch Centrum
BIG	Brain Imaging Genetics
BMI	Body mass index
BrainSCALE	Brain Structure and Cognition: an Adolescence Longitudinal twin study
BTEC	Business and Technology Education Council
CAMH	Centre for Addiction and Mental Health
CBASP	Cognitive Behavioral Analysis System of Psychotherapy
CBCL	Childhood behavior checklist
CCA	Canonical correlation analysis
CEG	Cognitive-experimental and Genetic study of ADHD and Control Sibling Pairs
CIAM	Cortical Inhibition and Attentional Modulation study
CLiNG	Clinical Neuroscience Göttingen
CM	Contrast mode
CSE	Certificate of Secondary Education
DALY	Disability adjusted life-years
DAWBA	Development and Well-being Assessment
DMN	Default Mode Network

DWI   Diffusion weighted imaging

ENIGMA   Enhancing Neuroimaging Genetics Through Meta-analysis

ESPAD   European School Survey Project on Alcohol and Other Drugs

EUROTRAIN European-Wide Investigation and Training Network on the Etiology and

Pathophysiology of Gilles de la Tourette Syndrome

FA   Fractional anisotropy

FBIRN Function Biomedical Informatics Research Network

FDR   False discovery rate

FIDMAG   Fundación para la Investigación y Docencia Maria Angustias Giménez

FIGS   Family Interview for Genetic Studies

FM   Functional mode

FP   Fractional Polynomial

GAIC   Generalized Akaike Information Criterion

GAMLSS   Generalised Additive Models for Location, Scale and Shape

GCSE   General Certificate of Secondary Education

GNVC   General National Vocational Qualification

GSP   Brain Genomics Superstruct Project

HMS   Homburg Multidiagnosis Study

HUBIN   Human Brain Informatics

ICV   Intracranial volume

IMH   Institute of Mental Health

IMpACT   The International Multicentre persistent ADHD Genetics Collaboration

KaSP	The Karolinska Schizophrenia Project
LEQ	Life Events Questionnaire
LMS	Lambda (λ), Mu (μ), Sigma (σ) (LMS)
MAS	Memory and Ageing Study
MCIC	MIND Clinical Imaging Consortium
MD	Mean diffusivity
MHRC	Mental Health Research Center
MM	Morphometry mode
MRI	Magnetic Resonance Imaging
NCNG	Norwegian Cognitive NeuroGenetics sample
NESDA	The Netherlands Study of Depression and Anxiety
NTR	Netherlands Twin Register
NU	Northwestern University
NUIG	National University of Ireland Galway
NVQ	National Vocational Qualification
NYU	New York University
OATS	Older Australian Twins Study
PCA	Principal component analysis
PING	Pediatric Imaging, Neurocognition and Genetics
QTIM	Queensland Twin Imaging
sCCA	Sparse canonical correlation analysis
RD	Radial diffusivity

rs-fMRI	Resting state functional connectivity
RSN	Resting state network
SD	Standard deviation
SHIP	Study of Health in Pomerania
sMRI	Structural magnetic tesonance imaging
Staged-Dep	Stages of Depression Study
SURPS	Substance Use Risk Profile Scale
TCI	Temperament and Character Inventory
TOP	Tematisk Område Psykoser (Thematically Organized Psychosis Research)
UMCU	Universitair Medisch Centrum Utrecht
UNIBA	University of Bari Aldo Moro
UPENN	University of Pennsylvania
WISC-IV	Wechsler Intelligence Scale for Children-IV
WMM	White matter mode
YLD	Years lost to disability

Chapter 1: Introduction

1.1   Adolescence as a Major Window of Vulnerability and Opportunity

According to the World Health Organization, there are 1.2 billion adolescents aged 10–19 years old, comprising 16.4% of the world's population [1]. Half of all mental illnesses begin before age 14. The top three causes of years lost to disability (YLD) lost among adolescents worldwide are neuropsychiatric disorders (45%), unintentional injuries (12%), and infectious diseases (10%) [2]. Disability adjusted life-years (DALY) rates are 12% higher in girls than in boys between 15 and 19 years [2]; moreover, amongst neuropsychiatric disorders, affective disorders appear to be on the rise, particularly in girls and young women [3]. However, this type of data does not take into account the full adolescence experience that can affect or be affected by neurodevelopment and risk for mental illness, such as pubertal development, temperament, psychological well-being, family and social environment, drug use, or school performance [3]. Childhood and adolescence therefore present a unique window of vulnerability to mental illness but also a window of opportunity to targeted and neuroscience-informed interventions to prevent or mitigate the risk of full-blown mental disorders [4,5].

To facilitate progress in the field it is critical that we focus on two research priorities:

1.2 Normative Centile Curves (Growth Curves)

Childhood and adolescence are periods of substantial neural reorganization, triggered in part by genetic and epigenetic factors, biological events related to the onset of puberty and by the changing social roles of young people [6-8]. Work in animals, as well as neuroimaging studies in humans, suggest that pubertal development corresponds with significant changes in the brains' structural and functional organization [9]. Despite these advances in knowledge at present the field lacks robust evidence for the age-related trajectories of brain phenotypes. In most fields in medicine, age-related trajectories derived from healthy individuals are routinely used as reference to identify deviations from the expected range, which are then used to trigger further investigations or interventions. A classic example is age-trajectory of body mass index (BMI) that has been instrumental in informing scientific models and public health policies relating to cardio-metabolic health [10]. To move forward, the field requires coordinated international initiatives to pool together data already acquired in population-based samples to derive age-related trajectories of key brain phenotypes.

1.3 Linking Brain Developmental Profiles to Psychopathological Traits, Cognition and the Environment

Previous studies have shown age related changes in brain morphometry that occur in parallel with the emergence of psychopathological traits [11]. However, a principled and comprehensive characterization of the link between developmental brain changes and psychopathology is still missing. Given that traits occur on a spectrum, of great importance is the characterization of how traits within the general population relate to brain development. In other words, studying what is normal becomes an essential part of what is defined and studied as abnormal. Patterns of structural correlates of traits in the pathological side of the spectrum can then be used to find at risk populations and suggest targets for intervention. Furthermore, early life experience and environment (particularly socioeconomic status, perinatal exposures, and traumatic events/life experiences) have long been linked to psychopathological outcomes [12-14]. The relation between the two and their interaction with brain development have been studied mostly in isolation and there has been little attempt to perform an all-encompassing synthesis of how environment relates to psychopathological traits in the context of brain development. It is important that we bridge this critical gap in knowledge to advance a biologically informed understanding of human psychopathology and will ultimately lend itself to targeted interventions for prevention or early detection of adverse adult mental health outcomes.

1.4 Research Objectives of Doctoral Thesis

1.4.1 To characterize normative brain changes across the lifespan in general population

1.4.2 To investigate the multivariate patterns of association between brain organization and psychopathological traits, cognition, and environment in adolescence

The preliminary findings from these studies are expected to inform future mechanistic and clinical studies in adolescent population, with an ultimate goal of biomarker discovery and risk stratification.

1.5 Summary of Doctoral Work

The current doctoral dissertation is comprised of four papers (two first author, one co-first author, and one second author) published by the candidate[15-18]. Each research objective has been investigated in two papers. In the first two papers published as a part of the Enhancing Neuro Imaging Genetics through Meta-Analysis (ENIGMA) consortium lifespan working group[15,16], the trajectories of brain cortical and subcortical structures were studied and centile curves for more than 17,000 individuals ages 3-90 are estimated. This work is now being pursued further to study the underlying mechanisms of normative changes, and its clinical implications. In the second set of papers[17,18], the candidate looks at the patterns of covariation between adolescent brain and multiple physical, cognitive, behavioral, and environmental factors in two large-scale neurodevelopmental cohorts, the European IMAGEN and the American Adolescent Brain and Cognitive Development (ABCD) study. This line of work has informed multiple projects on the relationship between brain and behavior and a personalized integrative approach to identifying individuals at risk of poorer outcomes. Each paper is briefly summarized below and then presented in full, representing the body of this Dissertation.

1.5.1 Cortical thickness across the lifespan: Data from 17,075 healthy individuals aged 3-90 years (Frangou, Modabbernia*, et al, Human Brain Mapping 2021)*

Previous research has shown that robust estimates of the association between age and brain morphometry require large-scale studies. In response, we used cross-sectional data from 17,075 individuals aged 3-90 years from the ENIGMA Consortium to investigate age-related changes in cortical thickness in 68 brain regions. We used fractional polynomial (FP) regression to quantify the nonlinear association between age and cortical thickness, and we computed normalized growth centiles using the parametric Lambda, Mu, and Sigma method. We estimated interindividual variability using meta-analysis and one-way analysis of variance. We observed that for most regions, their highest cortical thickness value was observed in childhood. Age and cortical thickness showed a negative association; the slope was steeper up to the third decade of life and more gradual thereafter; notable exceptions to this general pattern were entorhinal, temporopolar, and anterior cingulate cortices. Interindividual variability was largest in temporal and frontal regions across the lifespan. Age and its FP combinations explained up to 59% variance in cortical thickness. This is the largest study to date that to investigate cortical thickness trajectories across lifespan and may form the basis of further investigation on normative deviation in cortical thickness and its significance for behavioral and cognitive outcomes.

1.5.2 Subcortical volumes across the lifespan: Data from 18,605 healthy individuals aged 3-90 years (Dima, Modabbernia, et al, Human Brain Mapping 2021)

We capitalized on the resources of the ENIGMA Consortium to examine age-related trajectories inferred from cross-sectional measures of the ventricles, the basal ganglia (caudate, putamen, pallidum, and nucleus accumbens), the thalamus, hippocampus and amygdala using magnetic resonance imaging data obtained from 18,605 individuals aged 3-90 years. All subcortical structure volumes were at their maximum value early in life. The volume of the basal ganglia showed a monotonic negative association with age thereafter; there was no significant association between age and the volumes of the thalamus, amygdala and the hippocampus (with some degree of decline in thalamus) until the sixth decade of life after which they also showed a steep negative association with age. The lateral ventricles showed continuous enlargement throughout the lifespan. Age was positively associated with inter-individual variability in the hippocampus and amygdala and the lateral ventricles. These results were robust to potential confounders and could be used to examine the functional significance of deviations from typical age-related morphometric patterns.

1.5.3 Linked patterns of biological and environmental covariation with brain structure in adolescence: a population-based longitudinal study (Modabbernia, et al, Molecular Psychiatry 2020)

In this study, we sought to discover linked patterns of covariation between brain structural development and a wide array of these factors by leveraging data from the IMAGEN study, a longitudinal population-based cohort of adolescents. Brain structural measures and a comprehensive array of non-imaging features (relating to demographic, anthropometric, and psychosocial characteristics) were available on 1476 IMAGEN participants aged 14 years and from a subsample reassessed at age 19 years (n = 714). We applied sparse canonical correlation analyses (sCCA) to the cross-sectional and longitudinal data to extract modes with maximum covariation between neuroimaging and non-imaging measures. Separate sCCAs for cortical thickness, cortical surface area and subcortical volumes confirmed that each imaging phenotype was correlated with non-imaging features (sCCA r range: 0.30-0.65, all PFDR < 0.001). Total intracranial volume and global measures of cortical thickness and surface area had the highest canonical cross-loadings ($|\varrho|$ = 0.31-0.61). Age, physical growth and sex had the highest association with adolescent brain structure ($|\varrho|$ = 0.24-0.62); at baseline, further significant positive associations were noted for cognitive measures while negative associations were observed at both time points for prenatal parental smoking, life events, and negative affect and substance use in youth ($|\varrho|$ = 0.10-0.23). Sex, physical growth and age are the dominant influences on adolescent brain development. We highlight the persistent negative influences of prenatal parental smoking and youth substance use as they are modifiable and of relevance for public health initiatives.

1.5.4 Multivariate Patterns of Brain-Behavior-Environment Associations in the Adolescent Brain and Cognitive Development Study (Modabbernia, et al, Biological Psychiatry 2021)

In this work, we aimed to characterize how variation in adolescent structural and functional brain organization relates to behavioral, psychosocial, and environmental influences at the time of transition to adolescence. We used principal component analysis together with canonical correlation analysis to discover distinct patterns of covariation between measures of brain organization (brain morphometry, intracortical myelination, white matter integrity, and resting-state functional connectivity) and individual, psychosocial, and environmental factors in a nationally representative U.S. sample of 9623 individuals (aged 9-10 years, 49% female) participating in the ABCD study. These analyses identified 14 reliable modes of brain-behavior-environment covariation (canonical $r_{discovery}$ = .21 to .49, canonical r_{test} = .10 to .39, $p_{false\ discovery\ rate\ corrected}$ < .0001). Across modes, neighborhood environment, parental characteristics, quality of family life, perinatal history, cardiometabolic health, cognition, and psychopathology had the most consistent and replicable associations with multiple measures of brain organization; positive and negative exposures converged to form patterns of psychosocial advantage or adversity. These showed modality-general, respectively positive or negative, associations with brain structure and function with little evidence of regional specificity. Nested within these cross-modal patterns were more specific associations between prefrontal measures of morphometry, intracortical myelination, and functional connectivity with affective psychopathology, cognition, and family environment. In summary, we identified clusters of exposures that showed consistent modality-general associations with global measures of brain organization. These findings underscore the importance of understanding the complex and intertwined influences on brain organization and mental function during development and have the potential to inform public health policies aiming toward interventions to improve mental well-being.

Chapter 2: Cortical Thickness Across the Lifespan: Data from 17,075 Healthy Individuals Aged 3-90 Years

Originally published as:

Sophia Frangou#, Amirhossein Modabbernia#, Steven CR Williams, Efstathios Papachristou, Gaelle E. Doucet, Ingrid Agartz, Moji Aghajani et al. "Cortical thickness across the lifespan: Data from 17,075 healthy individuals aged 3–90 years." Hum Brain Mapp. 2021 Feb 17. doi: 10.1002/hbm.25364

#Contributed equally.

2.1 Study 1 Introduction

In the last two decades, there has been a steady increase in the number of studies of age-related changes in brain morphometry [11,19-35] as a means to understand the genetic and environmental influences on the human brain [34,36,37]. Here we focus specifically on cortical thickness, as assessed using magnetic resonance imaging (MRI), because this measure has established associations with behaviour and cognition in healthy populations [36,38-42] and with disease mechanisms implicated in neuropsychiatric disorders [43-53].

Structural MRI is the most widely used neuroimaging method in research and clinical settings because of its excellent safety profile, even in repeat administration, ease of data acquisition and high patient acceptability. Thus, establishing the typical patterns of age-related trajectories in cortical thickness could be a significant first step in the translational application of neuroimaging. The value of reference data is firmly established in medicine where deviations from the expected range are used to trigger further investigations or interventions. Classic examples are the growth charts developed by the World Health Organization (http://www.who.int/childgrowth/en/) and US National Center for Health Statistics (https://www.cdc.gov/growthcharts/cdc_charts.htm) to monitor child development and the body mass index (BMI) which has been instrumental in informing scientific models and public health policies relating to cardio-metabolic health [10].

There is significant uncertainty about the shape and inter-individual variability of age-related trajectories. Prior studies have reported linear and non-linear associations between age and cortical thickness (e.g., [23,24,26,28,35,41,42,54-58] that may be influenced by sex [59-61]. The present study harnesses the power of the Enhancing Neuroimaging Genetics through Meta-Analysis (ENIGMA) Consortium, a multinational collaborative network of researchers organized into working groups that conduct large-scale analyses integrating data from over 250 institutions [62-64]. Within ENIGMA, the focus of the Lifespan Working group is to delineate age-related trajectories of brain morphometry extracted from MRI images using standardized protocols and unified quality control procedures harmonized and validated across all participating sites. Moreover, the ENIGMA Lifespan dataset is the largest sample of healthy individuals available worldwide that offers the most comprehensive coverage of the human lifespan. This distinguishes the ENIGMA Lifespan dataset from other imaging samples, such as the UK Biobank (http://www.ukbiobank.ac.uk) which only includes individuals over 40 years of age. In the present study, we used MRI data from 17,075 healthy participants aged 3-90 years to define age-related trajectories and centile values for regional cortical thickness in the entire sample and for each sex. We estimated regional inter-individual variability it represents a major source of inter-study variation on age-related effects [61,65]. Based on prior literature our initial hypotheses were that cortical thickness in most regions will have an inverse U-shape trajectory with variable rates of decline between late childhood and old age that would be influenced by sex.

2.2 Study 1 Methods

2.2.1 Study Samples

De-identified demographic and cortical thickness data from 83 worldwide samples (Figure 1) were pooled to create the dataset used in this study. The pooled sample comprised 17,075 subjects (52% female) aged 3-90 years (Table 1). All sample participants had been screened to exclude psychiatric disorders, medical and neurological morbidity and cognitive impairment. Information about the screening protocols and eligibility criteria is provided in Supplemental Table S1.

Table 2.1. Characteristics of the included samples

Sample	Age, Mean, Years	Age, SD, Years	Age Range		Sample Size, N	Number of Males	Number of Females
ADHD NF	14	0.7	13	14	3	1	2
AMC	23	3.4	17	32	99	65	34
Barcelona 1.5T	15	1.9	11	17	24	10	14
Barcelona 3T	15	2.2	11	17	31	13	18
Betula	62	12.4	26	81	231	105	126
BIG 1.5T	28	14.3	13	82	1319	657	662
BIG 3T	24	8.1	18	71	1291	553	738
BIL&GIN	27	7.7	18	57	452	220	232
Bonn	39	6.5	29	50	175	175	0
BRAINSCALE	10	1.4	9	15	172	102	70
BRCATLAS	40	17.2	18	84	163	84	79
CAMH	44	19.3	18	86	141	72	69
Cardiff	26	7.8	18	58	265	78	187
CEG	16	1.8	13	19	31	31	0
CIAM	27	4.2	19	34	24	13	11
CLING	25	5.3	18	58	323	132	191
CODE	40	13.3	20	64	72	31	41
COMPULS/TS Eurotrain	11	1	9	13	42	29	13
Edinburgh	24	2.9	19	31	55	20	35
ENIGMA-HIV	25	4.3	19	33	30	16	14
ENIGMA-OCD (AMC/Huyser)	14	2.8	9	17	6	2	4
ENIGMA-OCD (IDIBELL)	33	10.4	20	50	20	8	12
ENIGMA-OCD (Kyushu/Nakao)	45	14.1	24	64	16	6	10
ENIGMA-OCD (London Cohort/Mataix-Cols)	38	11.6	26	63	10	2	8
ENIGMA-OCD (van den Heuvel 1.5T)	41	12.9	26	50	3	0	3
ENIGMA-OCD (van den Heuvel 3T)	36	10.9	22	55	8	4	4
ENIGMA-OCD-3T-CONTROLS	32	11	20	56	17	4	13
FBIRN	37	11.4	19	60	164	117	47
FIDMAG	38	10.1	19	64	123	54	69
GSP	27	16.5	18	90	2008	893	1115

HMS	40	12.2	19	64	55	21	34
HUBIN	42	8.8	19	56	102	69	33
IDIVAL (1)	65	9.8	49	87	34	13	21
IDIVAL (3)	30	7.8	19	50	104	63	41
IDIVAL(2)	28	7.6	15	52	80	50	30
IMAGEN	14	0.4	13	16	1722	854	868
IMH	32	9.8	20	58	73	48	25
IMpACT-NL	36	12.1	19	62	91	27	64
Indiana 1.5T	62	11.7	37	84	49	9	40
Indiana 3T	27	19.7	6	87	199	95	104
Johns Hopkins	44	12.5	20	65	85	42	43
KaSP	27	5.7	20	43	32	15	17
Leiden	17	4.8	8	29	572	279	293
MAS	79	4.7	70	90	385	176	209
MCIC	32	12.1	18	60	91	61	30
Melbourne	20	2.9	15	25	70	39	31
METHCT	27	6.5	19	53	39	29	10
MHRC	22	3.1	16	27	27	27	0
Muenster	35	12.1	17	65	744	323	421
NCNG	51	16.9	19	80	345	110	235
NESDA	40	9.7	21	56	65	23	42
NeuroIMAGE	17	3.4	9	27	252	115	137
Neuroventure	14	0.6	12	15	137	62	75
NTR (1)	15	1.4	11	18	37	14	23
NTR (2)	34	10.4	19	57	112	42	70
NTR (3)	30	5.9	20	42	29	11	18
NU	33	14.8	14	68	79	46	33
NUIG	36	11.5	18	58	92	53	39
NYU	31	8.7	19	52	51	31	20
OATS (1)	71	5.6	65	84	80	53	27
OATS (2)	69	5.1	65	81	13	7	6
OATS (3)	69	4	65	81	116	64	52
OATS (4)	70	4.7	65	89	90	63	27
Olin	36	13	21	87	582	231	351
Oxford	16	1.4	14	19	37	18	19
PING	12	4.8	3	21	431	223	208
QTIM	23	3.3	16	30	308	96	212
Sao Paolo (1)	28	6.1	17	43	51	32	19
Sao Paolo (3)	31	7.6	18	50	58	30	28
SCORE	25	4.3	19	39	44	17	27
SHIP 2	55	12.3	31	88	306	172	134
SHIP TREND	50	13.7	22	81	628	355	273
StagedDep	48	8.1	32	59	23	7	16

Stanford	45	12.6	21	61	8	4	4
STROKEMRI	45	22.1	18	78	52	19	33
Sydney	39	22.1	12	84	157	65	92
TOP	35	9.9	18	73	303	159	144
Tuebingen	40	12.4	24	61	38	12	26
UMCU 1.5T	33	12.5	17	66	278	158	120
UMCU 3T	44	14	19	78	144	69	75
UNIBA	27	9.1	18	63	130	67	63
UPENN	37	13.1	18	85	115	42	73
Yale	14	2.7	10	18	12	5	7
Total	31	18.2	3	90	17075	8212	8863

N=number; SD= standard deviation

Abbreviations of studies: ADHD-NF = Attention Deficit Hyperactivity Disorder-Neurofeedback Study; AMC = Amsterdam Medisch Centrum; Basel = University of Basel; Barcelona = University of Barcelona; Betula = Swedish longitudinal study on aging, memory, and dementia; BIG = Brain Imaging Genetics; BIL&GIN = a multimodal multidimensional database for investigating hemispheric specialization; Bonn = University of Bonn; BrainSCALE=Brain Structure and Cognition: an Adolescence Longitudinal twin study; CAMH = Centre for Addiction and Mental Health; Cardiff = Cardiff University; CEG = Cognitive-experimental and Genetic study of ADHD and Control Sibling Pairs; CIAM = Cortical Inhibition and Attentional Modulation study; CLiNG = Clinical Neuroscience Göttingen; CODE = formerly Cognitive Behavioral Analysis System of Psychotherapy (CBASP) study; Edinburgh = The University of Edinburgh; ENIGMA-HIV = Enhancing NeuroImaging Genetics through Meta-Analysis-Human Immunodeficiency Virus Working Group; ENIGMA-OCD = Enhancing NeuroImaging Genetics through Meta-Analysis-Obsessive Compulsive Disorder Working Group; FBIRN = Function Biomedical Informatics Research Network; FIDMAG = Fundación para la Investigación y Docencia Maria Angustias Giménez; GSP = Brain Genomics Superstruct Project; HMS = Homburg Multidiagnosis Study; HUBIN = Human Brain Informatics; IDIVAL = Valdecilla Biomedical Research Institute; IMAGEN = the IMAGEN Consortium; IMH=Institute of Mental Health, Singapore; IMpACT = The International Multicentre persistent ADHD Genetics Collaboration; Indiana = Indiana University School of Medicine; Johns Hopkins = Johns Hopkins University; KaSP= The Karolinska Schizophrenia Project; Leiden = Leiden University; MAS = Memory and Ageing Study; MCIC = MIND Clinical Imaging Consortium formed by the Mental Illness and Neuroscience Discovery (MIND) Institute now the Mind Research Network; Melbourne = University of Melbourne; Meth-CT = study of methamphetamine users, University of Cape Town; MHRC = Mental Health Research Center; Muenster = Muenster University; NESDA = The Netherlands Study of Depression and Anxiety; NeuroIMAGE = Dutch part of the International Multicenter ADHD Genetics (IMAGE) study; Neuroventure: the imaging part of the Co-Venture Trial funded by the Canadian Institutes of Health Research (CIHR); NCNG = Norwegian Cognitive NeuroGenetics sample; NTR = Netherlands Twin Register; NU = Northwestern University; NUIG = National University of Ireland Galway; NYU = New York University; OATS = Older Australian Twins Study; Olin = Olin Neuropsychiatric

2.2.2 Image acquisition and processing

Prior to pooling the data used in this study, researchers at each participating institution (a) used the ENIGMA MRI analysis protocols, which are based on FreeSurfer (http://surfer.nmr.mgh.harvard.edu) [66,67], to extract cortical thickness of 68 regions from high-resolution T1-weighted MRI brain scans collected at their site; (b) inspected all images by overlaying the cortical parcellations on the participants' anatomical scans; (c) excluded improperly segmented scans and outliers identified using five median absolute deviations (MAD) of that of the median value. Information on scanner vendor, magnetic field strengths, FreeSurfer version and acquisition parameters for each of the sample provided by the participating institutions is detailed in Supplemental Table S1.

2.2.3 Analysis of age-related trajectories in cortical thickness

We modelled the effect of age on regional cortical thickness using higher order fractional polynomial (FP) regression analyses [68,69] implemented in STATA software version 14.0 (Stata Corp., College Station, TX). FP regression is one of the most flexible methods to study the effect of continuous variables on a response variable [68,69]. FP allows for testing a broad family of shapes and multiple turning points while simultaneously

providing a good fit at the extremes of the covariates [68]. Prior to FP regression analysis,

cortical thickness values were harmonized between sites using the ComBat method in R

[70,71]. Originally developed to adjust for batch effect in genetic studies, ComBat uses an

empirical Bayes to adjust for inter-site (inter-scanner) variability in the data, while We

centred each brain region so that the intercept of an FP was zero for all covariates. We

used a predefined set of power terms (-2, -1, -0.5, 0.5, 1, 2, 3) and the natural logarithm

function, and up to four power combinations to identify the best fitting model. FP for age

is written as $\text{age}^{(p1,p2,\dots p6)\prime}\beta$ where p in $\text{age}^{(p1,p2,\dots p6)}$ refers to regular powers except $\text{age}^{(0)}$

which refers to ln(age). Powers can be repeated in FP and each time it is repeated it is

multiplied by another ln(age). As an example

$$\text{age}^{(0,1,1)\prime}\beta = \beta_0 + \beta_1 \text{age}^0 + \beta_2 \text{age}^1 + \beta_3 \text{age}^1 \ln(\text{age})$$

$$= \beta_0 + \beta_1 \ln(\text{age}) + \beta_2 \text{age} + \beta_3 \text{age} \ln(\text{age})$$

494 models were trained for each region. Model comparison was performed using a

partial F-test and the lowest degree model with a non-significant P-value was selected as the optimal model. Critical alpha value was set at 0.01 to decrease the probability of over-

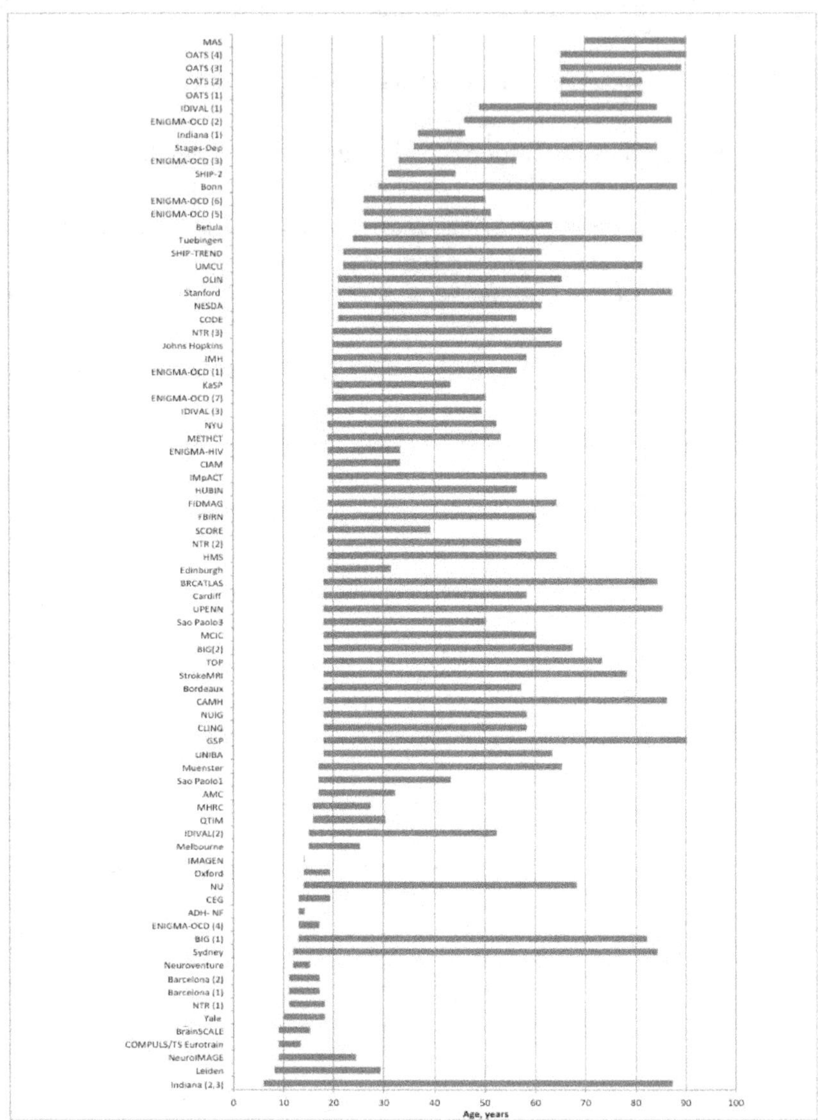

Figure 2.1. Age range for each sample
Abbreviations are explained in Table 1 and further details of each sample are provided in the supplemental material.

fitting. The age at maximum cortical thickness for each cortical region was the maximum fitted value of the corresponding optimal FP model.

Further, we divided the dataset in three age-groups corresponding to early (3-29 years), middle (30-59 years) and late life (60-90 years). Within each age-group, we calculated Pearson's correlation coefficient between age and regional cortical thickness. Finally, we used the *cocor* package (version 1.1-3) in R to obtain P-values for the differences in correlation coefficient between males and females in each age-group.

2.2.4 Inter-individual Variation in Cortical Thickness

The residuals of the FP regression models for each cortical region were normally distributed. Using one-way analysis of variance, we extracted the residual variance around the optimal fitted FP regression model so as to identify age-group differences in inter-individual variation for each cortical region. Separately for each age-group (t), we calculated the mean variance of each cortical region using $\left(\dfrac{\sum \sqrt{e_i^2}}{n_t}\right)$ where e^2 denotes the squared residual variance of that region around the best fitting FP regression line for each individual (i) of that age-group, and n the number of observations in that age-group. Because the square root of the squared residuals was positively skewed, we applied a natural logarithm transformation to the calculated variance. To account for multiple comparisons (68 regions assessed in three age-groups), statistical inference was based on a Bonferroni adjusted *p*-value of 0.0007 as a cut-off for a significant *F*-test.

To confirm that the sample effect did not drive the inter-individual variability

analyses, we also conducted a meta-analysis of the standard deviation of the regional

cortical thickness in each age-group, following previously validated methodology [72]. To

test whether inter-individual variability is a function of surface area (and possibly

measurement error by FreeSurfer) we plotted SD values of each region against their

corresponding average surface area.

2.2.5 Centile Values of Cortical Thickness

We calculated the centiles (0.4, 1, 2.5, 5, 10, 25, 50, 75, 90, 95, 97.5, 99, 99.6) for each

regional cortical thickness by sex and hemisphere as normalized growth centiles using

parametric Lambda (λ), Mu (μ), Sigma (σ) (LMS) method (Cole and Green, 1992) in the

Generalised Additive Models for Location, Scale and Shape (GAMLSS) package (version

5.2-0) in R (http://cran.r-project.org/web/packages/gamlss/index.html) [73,74]. LMS is

considered a powerful method for estimating centile curves based on the distribution of

a response variable at each covariate value (in this case age). GAMLSS uses a penalized

maximum likelihood function to estimate parameters of smoothness (effective degrees of

freedom) which are then used to estimate the λ, μ and σ parameters [75]. The goodness of

fit for these parameters in the GAMLSS algorithm is established by minimizing the

Generalized Akaike Information Criterion (GAIC) index.

2.3 Study 1 Results

2.3.1 Age-related trajectories in cortical thickness

Figure 2 shows characteristic trajectories for cortical regions in each lobe, while the

trajectories of all cortical regions are provided in Supplemental File S1.

In most regions, cortical thickness showed a steep decrease until 3rd decade of life

followed by monotonic gradual decline thereafter (Supplemental Table S2). However,

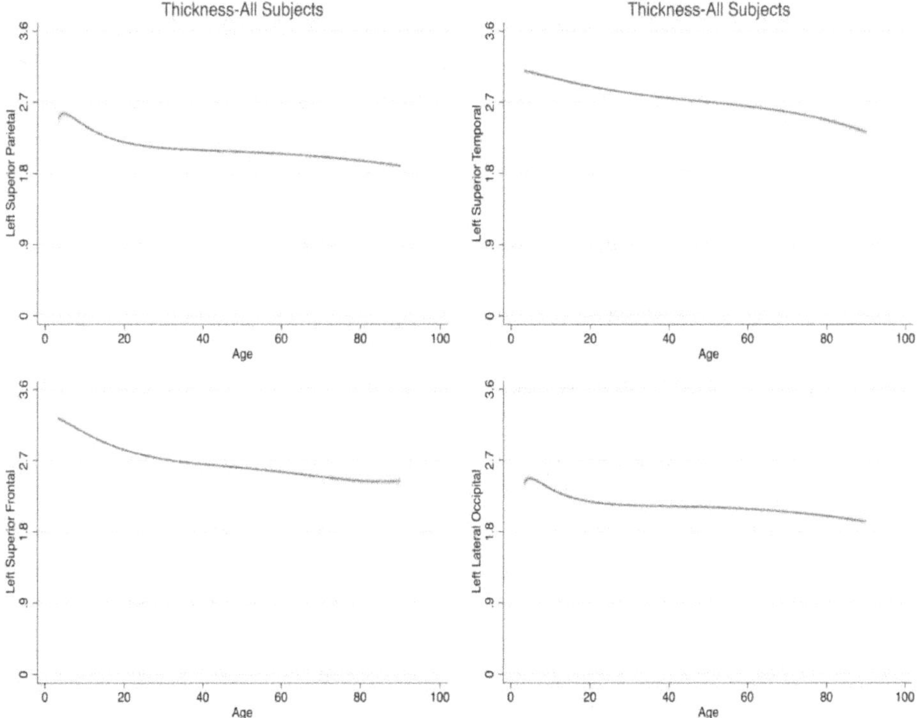

Figure 2.2. Illustrative age-related trajectories of cortical thickness
We present exemplars from each lobe as derived from fractional polynomial analyses of the
entire dataset. Age-related trajectories of thickness for all cortical regions (for the entire dataset
and separately for males and females) are given in the supplementary material.

both entorhinal and temporopolar cortices showed an inverse U relation with age

bilaterally while in the anterior cingulate cortex (ACC) cortical thickness showed an

attenuated U-shaped trajectory. In general, age and its FP combinations explained up to

59% of the variance in mean cortical thickness (Supplemental Table S2). Age explained the smallest proportion of the variance for entorhinal (1-2%) and temporopolar (2-3%) cortices, whereas it explained the largest proportion of variance for superior frontal and precuneus gyri (50-52%). We observed some significant sex differences in the slopes of age-related regional cortical thickness reduction. In general, in the early-life group (3-29 years), the slopes for mean cortical thickness were not meaningfully different for males (r=-0.59) than females (r=-0.56). Similarly, in the middle-life group (30-59 years) the slopes for mean cortical thickness were steeper for men (r =-0.39 to -0.38) than for women (r-range=-0.27). In the late-life group (61-90 years) there was no meaningful difference between men (r-range= -0.30 to -0.29) and women (r-range= =-0.33 to -0.31) because the slopes of regional cortical thickness reduction became less pronounced in men while slightly increasing in women. At the regional level, the slope of cortical thinning in the early-life group was greater (P<0.0007) in males than in females in the bilateral cuneus, lateral occipital, lingual, superior parietal, postcentral, and paracentral, precuneus, and pericalcarine gyri. In middle-life age-group, the slope of cortical thinning was greater (P<0.0002) in men than in women in the bilateral pars orbitalis and pars triangularis as well as left isthmus cingulate, pars opercularis, precuneus, rostral middle frontal, and supramarginal, and right fusiform, inferior temporal, inferior parietal, lateral occipital, lateral orbitofrontal, rostral anterior cingulate, superior frontal, supramarginal and

insula. (Figure 3, Supplemental Table S3, Supplemental Figure S1).

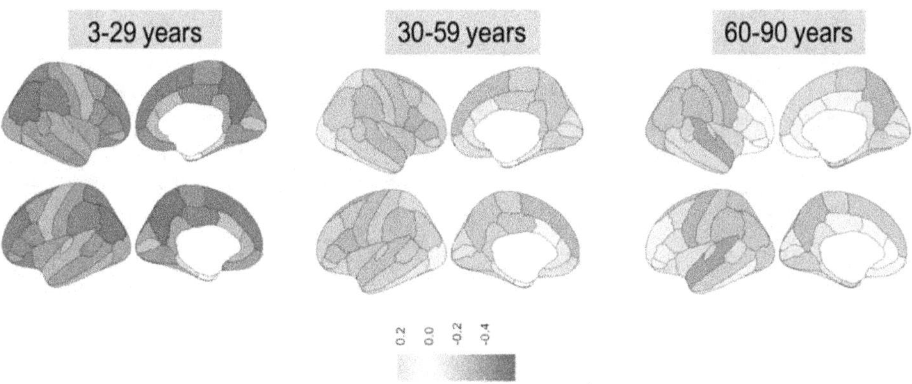

Figure 2.3. Correlation between age and cortical thickness across age-groups
Left panel: early life age-group (3-29 years); Middle panel: middle life age-group (30-59 years);
Right panel: late life age-group (60-90 years).

2.3.2 Inter-individual Variation in Cortical Thickness

Details of the inter-individual variation for all cortical regions in each group are

provided in Supplemental Table S4, Supplemental Figure S2, and Figure 4. Across age-

groups, the inter-individual variability in most cortical regions as measured by pooled

SD was between 0.1 and 0.2; Higher levels of inter-individual variation were also

observed but were mainly apparent bilaterally for the entorhinal, parahippocampal,

transverse temporal, temporopolar, frontopolar, anterior and isthmus of the cingulate

cortex, and the *pars orbitalis*. The meta-analysis conducted as per [72] confirmed the

replicability of these findings in each age-group (early, middle and late life). We observed

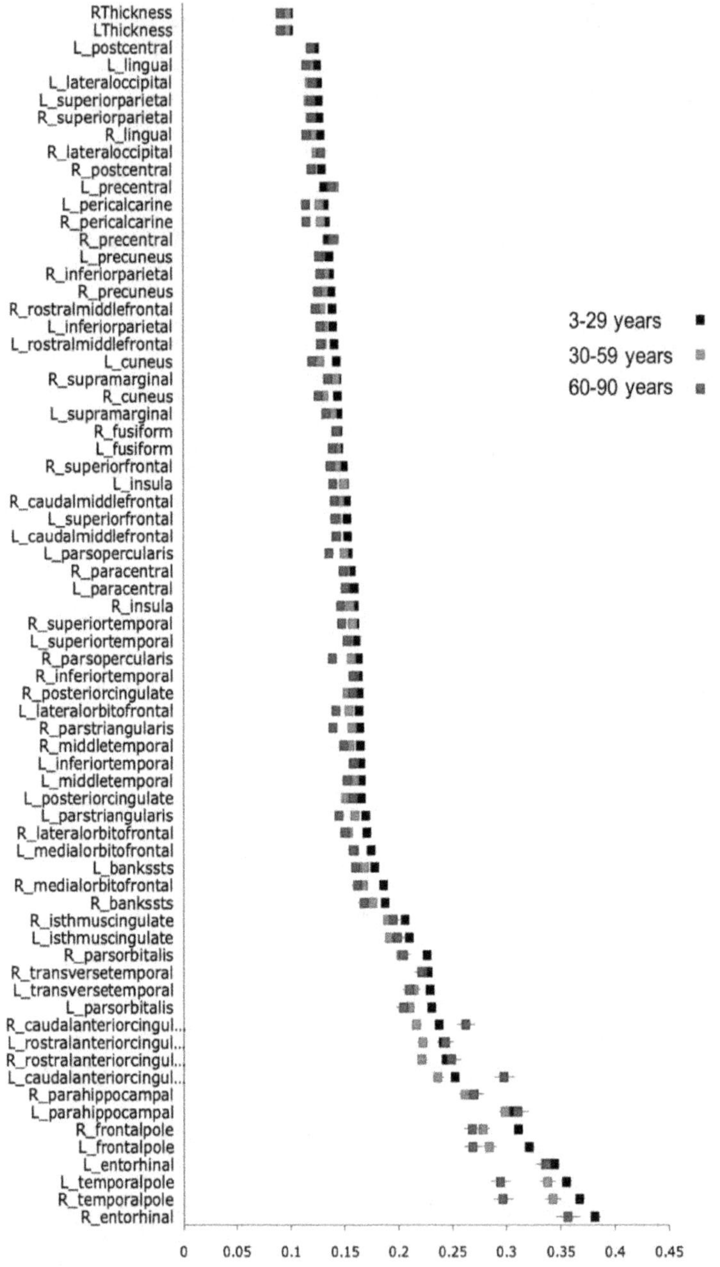

Figure 2.4. Meta-analysis of pooled standard deviation in the entire dataset

a nonlinear association between regional cortical surface area and inter-individual variability in that variability was typically higher in regions with smaller surface areas (Supplementary Figure S3).

2.3.3 Centile Curves of Cortical Thickness

Representative centiles curves for each lobe are presented in Figure 5. Centile values for the thickness of each cortical region stratified by sex and hemisphere are provided in Supplemental Table S5-Table S7 and Supplemental File S2.

2.4 Study 1 Discussion

In the present study, we provide the most comprehensive characterization of lifetime trajectories of regional cortical thickness based on multiple analytic methods (i.e., FP analysis, meta-analysis and centile calculations) and the largest dataset of cortical thickness measures available from healthy individuals aged 3 to 90 years. In addition to sample size, the study benefited from the standardized and validated protocols for data extraction and quality control that are common to all ENIGMA sites and have supported all published ENIGMA structural MRI studies [43,45,50,51].

As predicted, most regional cortical thickness reached its maximum value between 3-10 years of age, showed a steep decrease during the second and third decades of life and an attenuated or plateaued slope until later life. This pattern was independent of the hemisphere and sex. A recent review [34] has highlighted contradictions between studies that report an increase in cortical thickness during early childhood and studies that report

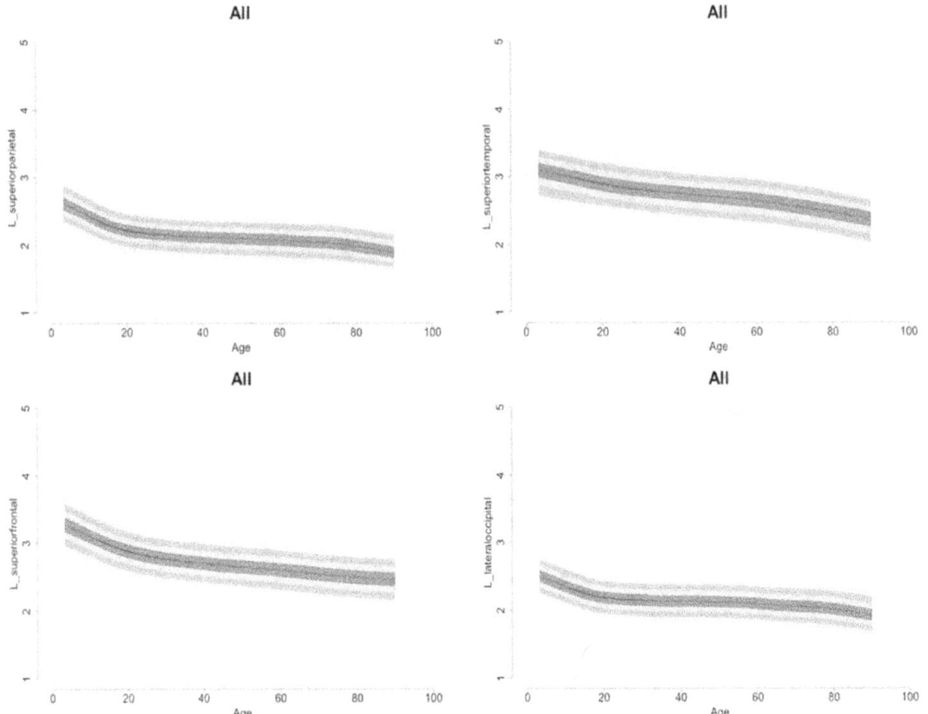

Figure 2.5. Illustrative Normative Centile Curves of Cortical Thickness
We present exemplars from each lobe as derived from LMS of the entire dataset. Normative Centile Curves of thickness for all cortical regions (for the entire dataset and separately for males and females) are given in the supplementary material.

a decrease in cortical thickness during the same period. The results from our large-scale analysis help reconcile previous findings as we show that the median age at maximum thickness for most cortical regions is in the lower bound of the age range we examined here.

In the entorhinal and temporopolar regions, cortical thickness remained largely stable until 7th-8th decades of life when it started to decline. Although the FreeSurfer estimation of cortical thickness in these regions is often considered suboptimal (compared to the rest of the brain), we note that our findings are consistent with a prior multicenter study of 1,660 healthy individuals [21]. Further, the current study supports results from the National Institute of Health MRI study of 384 individuals that found no significant change in the bilateral entorhinal and medial temporopolar cortex between the ages of 4-22 years [76]. A further study of 207 healthy adults aged 23-87 years also showed no significant cortical thinning in the entorhinal cortex until the 6th decade of life [30]. These observations suggest that the cortex of the entorhinal and temporopolar regions is largely preserved across the lifespan in healthy individuals. Both these regions are known to contribute to episodic memory and the temporopolar region is also involved in semantic memory [77-79]. Degenerative changes of the temporopolar cortex have been reliably associated with semantic dementia, which is characterized by loss of conceptual knowledge about real-world items [80]. The integrity and resting metabolic rate of the temporopolar cortex decrease with age [81-84], and lower perfusion rates in this region correlate with cognitive impairment in patients with Alzheimer's disease (AD) [85]. Entorhinal cortical thickness is a reliable marker of episodic memory performance [36,86] and entorhinal cortex volume and metabolism are reduced in patients with Alzheimer's Disease and mild cognitive impairment [39,86]. We therefore infer that "accelerated" entorhinal and temporopolar cortical thinning may be a marker of age-related cognitive decline; as they grow older, individuals at risk of cognitive decline may show a gradual shift in the distribution of the cortical thickness of these regions to the left which aligns with the exponential age-related increase in the incidence of AD in later decades of life [87].

The thickness of the ACC showed an attenuated U-shaped association with age. This observation replicates an earlier finding in 178 healthy individuals aged 7-87 years, which also found a U-shaped relationship between ACC thickness and age [27]. The U-shaped age trajectory of ACC thickness might explain divergent findings in previous studies that have reported age-related increases [25,88], age-related reductions or no change [19,33,36,76,89].

A consistently higher degree of inter-individual variation was observed in the most rostral frontal regions (frontopolar cortex and *pars orbitalis*), in the ACC and in several temporal regions (entorhinal, parahippocampal, temporopolar and transverse temporal cortex). To some degree, greater variability in several of these regions may reflect variability in measurement associated with their smaller size (Supplementary Figure S3). Nevertheless, the pattern observed suggests that greater inter-individual variability may be a feature of proisocortical and periallocortical regions (in the cingulate and temporal cortices) that are anatomically connected to prefrontal isocortical regions, and particularly the frontopolar cortex. This isocortical region of the prefrontal cortex is considered evolutionarily important based on its connectivity and function compared both to other human cortical regions and corresponding cortical regions in non-human primates [90,91]. The frontopolar region has several microstructural characteristics, such as higher number and width of minicolumns and greater inter-neuron space, which are conducive to facilitating neuronal connectivity [91]. According to the popular 'gateway' hypothesis, the lateral frontopolar cortex implements processing of external information ('stimulus-oriented' processing) while the medial frontopolar cortex attends to self-generated or maintained representations ("stimulus-independent" processing) [92]. Stimulus-oriented processing in the frontopolar cortex is focused on multitasking and goal-directed planning while stimulus-independent processing involves mainly mentalizing and social cognition [93]. The other regions (entorhinal, parahippocampal, cingulate, and temporopolar) with high inter-individual variation in cortical thickness are periallocortical and proisocortical regions that are functionally connected to the medial frontopolar cortex [93,94]. Notably, the periallocortex and proisocortex are considered transitional zones between the phylogenetically older allocortex and the more evolved isocortex [95]. Specifically, the entorhinal cortex is perialiocortical [96,97], the cingulate and parahippocampal cortices are proisocortical and the cortex of the temporopolar region is mixed [98,99]. Considered together, these regions are core nodes of the default mode network (DMN; [100]). At present, it is unclear whether this higher inter-individual variation in the cortical thickness of the DMN nodes is associated with functional variation, but this is an important question for future studies.

The results presented here are based on the largest available dataset worldwide covering the human lifespan. However, none of the pooled samples in the current study was longitudinal. We fully appreciate that longitudinal studies are considered preferable to cross-sectional designs when aiming to define age-related brain morphometric trajectories. However, a longitudinal study of this size over nine decades of life is not feasible. In addition to problems with participant recruitment and retention, such a lengthy study would have involved changes in scanner types, magnetic field strengths and acquisition protocols in line with necessary upgrades and technological advances. We took several steps to mitigate against site effects. First, we ensured that we used age-overlapping datasets throughout. Second, standardized analyses and quality control protocols were used to extract cortical thickness measures at all participating institutions. Third, we estimated and controlled for the contribution of site and scanner using ComBat prior to conducting our analysis. The validity of the findings reported here is reinforced by their alignment with the results from short-term longitudinal studies of cortical thickness [29-32,35,46]. The generalizability of our findings for the older age group is qualified by our selection of individuals who appear to be ageing successfully in terms of cognitive function and absence of significant medical morbidity. Nevertheless, despite the efforts to include only healthy older individuals, the observed pattern of brain aging may still be influenced by subclinical mental or medical conditions. For example, vascular risk factors (e.g., hypertension) are prevalent in older individuals and have been associated with decline in the age-sensitive regions identified here (Raz et al., 2005). Thus, we cannot conclusively exclude the possibility that such factors may have contributed to our results.

Cellular studies show that the number of neurons, the extent of dendritic arborization, and amount of glial support explain most of the variability in cortical thickness [38,47,101,102]. MRI lacks the resolution to assess microstructural tissue properties but provides an estimate of cortical thickness based on the MR signal [34]. Nevertheless, there is remarkable similarity between MRI-derived thickness maps and post-mortem data [29].

The findings of the current study suggest several avenues of further research. MRI-derived measures of cortical thickness do not provide information on the mechanisms that underlie the observed age-related trajectories. However, the centile values across the lifespan, provided here, could be used to study factors that may lead to deviations in cortical thickness way from the expected age-appropriate range. Such factors may be genetic, epigenetic, hormonal, socioeconomic or related to physical traits and health and lifestyle choices. Additionally, the results of the current study provide a new avenue for investigating the functional correlates, either cognitive or behavioral, of age-related changes and inter-individual variation in regional cortical thickness.

In summary, we performed a large-scale analysis using data from 17,075 individuals to investigate the lifespan trajectories of cortical thickness in healthy individuals. Our results may shed light on the uncertainties regarding age-related developmental trajectories for cortical thickness. Estimated centile values and inter-individual variability measures have the potential to provide scientists and clinicians with new tools to detect morphometric deviations and investigating associated

behavioral and cognitive phenotypes.

2.5 Study 1 Supplemental Material

Due to very large volume of the supplemental files, important tables and figures

are presented below and the rest are available only online. The full supplemental material

for this study can be accessed online through the following links

File 1.

https://onlinelibrary.wiley.com/action/downloadSupplement?doi=10.1002%2Fhbm.2536

4&file=hbm25364-sup-0001-Supinfo01.docx

This file includes the following figures and tables

Figure S1 Histogram of age-distribution across all samples

Figure S2. Correlation between age and cortical thickness across age-groups and

stratified by sex

Figure S3. Meta-analysis of pooled standard deviation stratified by sex

Figure S4. Pooled Standard deviation of cortical regions as a function of surface area

Table S1. Screening Process and Eligibility Criteria, Scanner, Image Acquisition

Parameters and Image Segmentation Software

Table S2. Variance Explained by Age in fractional polynomial model

Table S3: Pearson's Correlation Coefficient between Age and Cortical Thickness

Table S4. Interindividual variations in cortical thickness

Table S5. Centile Values for Cortical Thickness

Table S6. Centile Values for Cortical Thickness in Males

Table S7. Centile Values for Cortical Thickness in Females

<u>File 2.</u>

https://onlinelibrary.wiley.com/action/downloadSupplement?doi=10.1002%2Fhbm.2536
4&file=hbm25364-sup-0002-Supinfo02.pdf

This file includes the cortical thickness trajectories for all regions for all participants as

well as stratified by sex

<u>File 3.</u>

https://onlinelibrary.wiley.com/action/downloadSupplement?doi=10.1002%2Fhbm.2536
4&file=hbm25364-sup-0003-Supinfo03.pdf

This file includes the centile curves of cortical thickness for all regions for all participants

as well as stratified by sex

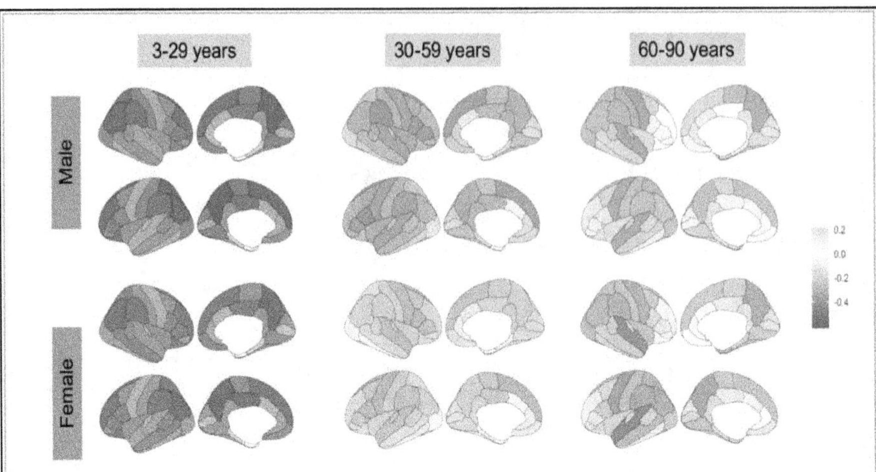

Figure S1. Correlation between age and cortical thickness across age-groups and stratified by sex

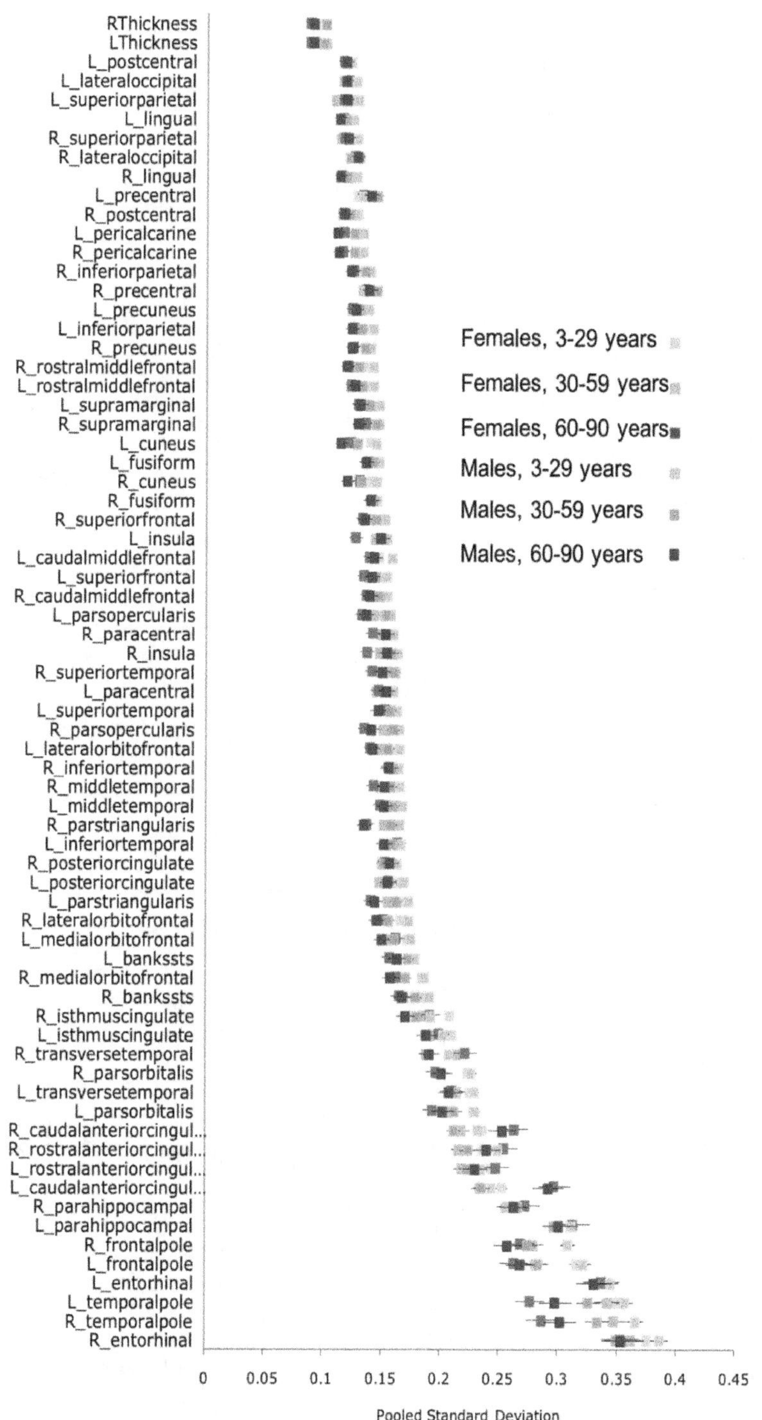

Figure S2. Meta-analysis of pooled standard deviation stratified by sex

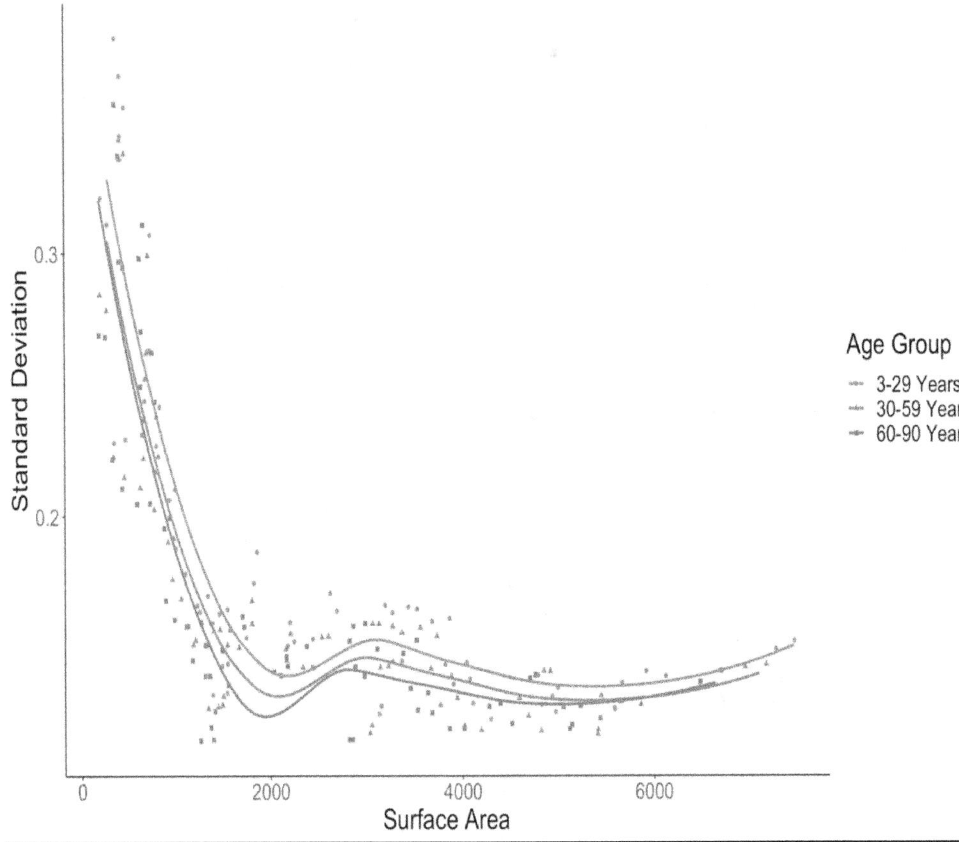

Figure S3. Pooled Standard deviation of cortical regions as a function of surface area

Table S1. Screening Process and Eligibility Criteria, Scanner, Image Acquisition Parameters and Image Segmentation Software

Sample	Screening Process	Eligibility Criteria	Magnet strength/ Scanner Vendor	Acquisition parameters	Free/S urfer version
ADHD-NF	KSADS	No head trauma, no neurological and psychiatric history, no lifetime alcohol or substance abuse, no previous or current use of psychotropic medication, IQ>75.	3T Siemens Tim Trio	T1-weighted 3D MPRAGE; TR/TE/TI/FA=2300ms/30 30ms/900ms/9°; Image matrix= 256 × 256; 192 sagittal slices; voxel size=1mm^3	5.3

AMC	Personal Interview	No head trauma, no medical, neurological or psychiatric history, no lifetime alcohol or substance abuse, no previous or current use of psychotropic medication, IQ>75. No history of any psychiatric disorders in 1st degree family members.	3T Philips Intera	T1-weighted 3D MPRAGE; TE range= 3.5-4.6ms, TR range= 9-9.663ms, FA=	5.1
Barcelona 1.5T	KSADS	No head trauma, no medical, neurological or psychiatric history, no lifetime alcohol or substance abuse, no previous or current use of psychotropic medication, IQ>75. No history of any psychiatric disorders in 1st degree family members.	1.5 T General Electric Signa	T1-weighted; image matrix = 256 x 256; 128 slices; voxel size 1 x 1 x 1 mm³.	5.3
Barcelona 3T	KSADS	No head trauma, no medical, neurological or psychiatric history, no lifetime alcohol or substance abuse, no previous or current use of psychotropic medication, IQ>75. No history of any psychiatric disorders in 1st degree family members.	3 T Siemens MAGNETOM TIM Trio	T1-weighted; image matrix = 256 x 256; 240 slices; voxel size 1 x 1 x 1 mm³.	5.3
Betula	Personal Interview	No head trauma, no medical, neurological or psychiatric history, no lifetime alcohol or substance abuse, no previous or current use of psychotropic medication.	3T General Electric Discovery MR750	T1-weighted MPRAGE; TR/TE/TI/FA=8.1240 ms/3.2000 ms/450ms/ 12°; image matrix = 256x256	5.3
BIG	Questionnaire for psychiatric history	No head trauma, no medical, neurological or psychiatric history, no lifetime alcohol or substance abuse, no previous or current use of psychotropic medication, IQ>70. No history of any psychiatric disorders in 1st or 2nd degree family members.	1,5 T Siemens Sonata and Avanto and 3 T Siemens Trio, TimTrio and Skyra	T1-weighted 3D MPRAGE; TR/TE/TI/sagittal slices = 1940-2730 ms/850-110 ms/2.92-4.58 ms; 176-192 sagittal slices; voxel size= 1.0x1.0x1.0 mm³	5.3
BIL&GIN	Personal Interview	No head trauma, no current neurological or psychiatric disorders, no current use of psychotropic medication, IQ>70.	3T Phillips ACHIEVA	T1 - weighted 3D; TR/TE/TI/FA=20 ms/4.6 ms/800ms/ 10°; turbo field echo factor = 65; sense factor = 2; matrix size = 256x256x180mm 3 ; voxel size= 1.0x1.0x1.0 mm³	5.3
Bonn	Personal interview	No head trauma, no medical, neurological or psychiatric history, no previous or current use of psychotropic medication.	3T Siemens Trio	TR/TE/FA= 1570-1660ms/2.75-3.42ms/8-9°	NA
BrainSCALE	Personal interview	No head trauma, no medical, neurological or psychiatric history, no lifetime alcohol or substance abuse, no previous or	1.5T Philips Achieva	T1-weighted 3D SPGR; TR/TE/ FA= 30 ms/4.6 ms/30°; image	5.1

		current use of psychotropic medication.		matrix=256x256; 160–180 contiguous coronal slices; voxel size=1 x 1 x 1.2 mm³	
BRCATLAS	Telephone interview	No head trauma, no medical, neurological or psychiatric history, no lifetime alcohol or substance abuse, no mild cognitive impairment, no previous or current use of psychotropic medication, IQ>75.	3T GE Signa	T1-weighted 3D; TR/TE/TI/FA= 6.9 ms/2.8 ms/650 ms/8°; Image matrix = 256 x 256 x 180mm³; voxel size=1mm³	
CAMH	SCID	No head trauma, no neurological or psychiatric history, no alcohol or substance abuse preceding 6 months, no previous or current use of psychotropic medication, IQ>75. No history of any psychotic disorders in 1st degree family members.	1.5 T GE (echospeed)	124 Axial inversion recovery–prepared spoiled gradient recall images, 1.5-mm-thick slice acquisition TE/TR/TI/FA=5.3ms/12.3 ms/300.0ms/20°.	5.3
Cardiff	MINI	No head trauma, no medical history, including neurological and psychiatric history, no alcohol or substance abuse in the preceding 6 months, no previous or current use of psychotropic medication.	3T General Electric Signa	T1-weighted 3D FSPGR; TR/TE/TI/FA=7.9ms/3.0 ms/450ms/20°; Image matrix= 256 × 192 x 172; voxel size=1mm³	5.3
CODE (1-5)	SCID	No head trauma, no medical, neurological or psychiatric history, no lifetime alcohol or substance abuse, no previous or current use of psychotropic medication, IQ>75. No history of any psychiatric disorders in 1st degree family members.	3T Siemens Trio (4 CODE sites); 3T Philips Achieva (1 CODE site)	Siemens: T1 mprage, 1mm isotropic voxels, 12 channel head coil, TR=1900ms, TE=2.52ms, 170/192 slices. Philips: T1 3D-TFE, 1mm isotropic voxels, 8 channel head coil, TR=8.3ms, TE=3.8ms, 170 slices	5.3
CEG	Teacher and parent Conners'	No head trauma, no medical history, including neurological and psychiatric history, no alcohol or substance abuse in the preceding 6 months, no previous or current use of psychotropic medication. IQ>75	3T General Electric Signa	T1-weighted 3D SPGR; TR/TE/ FA=2000ms/30ms/90°; Image matrix= 128 × 128; 43 slices	5.3
CIAM	SCID	No head trauma or psychiatric history, no previous or current use of psychotropic medication, IQ>75.	3T Siemens Allegra	T1-weighted 3D MPRAGE; TR/TE/TI/FA= 2530 ms/1.53, 3.21, 4.89, 6.57/2.91 ms/ ms/7°; image matrix= 256x256; 128 sagittal slices; voxel size= 1.3x1.0x1.3 mm³	5.3
CLiNG	Personal Interview	No head trauma, no medical, neurological or psychiatric history, no lifetime alcohol or	3T Siemens Tim Trio	T1-weighted 3D MPRAGE; TR/TE/TI/FA=2250	5.3

COMPULS/T S EUROTRAI N	KSADS	substance abuse, no previous or current use of psychotropic medication, IQ>75. No history of any psychiatric disorders in 1st degree family members. No head trauma, no medical, neurological or psychiatric history, no alcohol or substance abuse preceding 6 months, no previous or current use of psychotropic medication, IQ>75. No history of any psychiatric disorders in 1st or 2nd degree family members.	3T Siemens Tim Trio and Prisma	T1-weighted 3D MPRAGE; TR/TE/FA=2300 ms/2.98 ms/9°; image matrix = 256 x 256; 176 sagittal slices; voxel size= 1x1x1.2 mm³	5.3
Edinburgh	SCID-NP	No head trauma, no medical, neurological or psychiatric history, no previous or current use of psychotropic medication, IQ>75. No history of any psychiatric disorders in 1st and 2nd degree family members.	1.5T Siemens Magnetom Essenza 1.5T General Electric Signa	T1-weighted MPRAGE; TR/TE/TI/FA =10 ms/4 ms/200 ms/8o; 128 contiguous coronal slices; voxel size=1.25 x 1.25 x 1.20 mm T1-weighted MPRAGE; TR/TE/TI/FA =10 ms/4 ms/500 ms/8o; image matrix = 192 x 192; 180 coronal slices; voxel size=1.25 x 1.25 x 1.2 mm3	5.3
ENIGMA-HIV	MINI	No head trauma, no medical, neurological or psychiatric history, no alcohol or substance abuse preceding 6 months, no previous or current use of psychotropic medication, IQ>75. No mild cognitive impairment	3T Siemens Allegra	T1-weighted MPRAGE; TR/TE/TI/FA=2400 ms/2.38 ms/1000 ms/ 8°; 162 slices; voxel size= 1 mm³	5.1
ENIGMA-OCD (3T OCD control)	MINI-Plus	No head trauma, no medical, neurological or psychiatric history, no lifetime alcohol or substance abuse, no previous or current use of psychotropic medication, IQ>75. No cognitive impairment	3T Siemens Allegra	T1-weighted 3D MPRAGE; TR/TE/TI/FA=2300 ms/3.93 ms/ 1100 ms/12°; image matrix =256×240; 160 contiguous sagittal slices; voxel size=1.3 x 1 x 1 mm³	5.3
ENIGMA-OCD (van den Heuvel 1.5T)	SCID-I	No medical or psychiatric history	1.5T Siemens Sonata	T1-weighted 3D MPRAGE; TR/TE/TI/FA=2700 ms/4 ms/ 950 ms/8°; image matrix =256×192; 160 slices; voxel size= 1 mm³	5.3

ENIGMA-OCD (van den Heuvel 3T)	SCID-I	No medical or psychiatric history	3T General Electric Signa	T1-weighted 3D MPRAGE; image matrix =256×256; 172 slices; voxel size= 1x0.977x0.977 mm^3	5.3
ENIGMA-OCD (Huyser)	Personal Interview	No head trauma, no medical, neurological or psychiatric history, no lifetime alcohol or substance abuse, no previous or current use of psychotropic medication, IQ>75.	3T Phillips Intera	T1-weighted 3D MPRAGE; TR/TE/ FA=9.69 ms/4.60 ms/8°; image matrix =256×256; 182 slices; voxel size=1 x 1 x 1.2 mm^3	5.3
ENIGMA-OCD (Mataix-Cols)	SCID	No head trauma, no neurological or psychiatric history, no lifetime alcohol or substance abuse, no previous or current use of psychotropic medication, IQ>75.	1.5T General Electric Signa	T1-weighted 3D SPGR; TR/TE/FA= 14.8 ms/ 1.7 ms/ 20°; image matrix= 256 x 256 x 124; voxel size: 0.94 x 0.94 x 1.50 mm	5.3
ENIGMA-OCD (Nakao)	Personal Interview	No head trauma, no neurological or psychiatric history, no lifetime alcohol or substance abuse.	3T Phillips Achieva	T1-weighted 3D TFE; TR/TE/TI/FA=8.2 ms/3.8ms/1026 ms/8°; image matrix =240×240; 190 slices; voxel size=1 mm^3	5.3
ENIGMA-OCD (IDIBELL)	SCID-I/NP	No head trauma, no medical, neurological or psychiatric history, no alcohol or substance abuse in the preceding 6 months, no previous or current use of psychotropic medication, IQ>70. No history of any psychiatric disorders in 1st or 2nd degree family members	1.5 T General Electric Signa	T1-weighted 3D FSPGR; TR/TE/ FA=11.8ms/4.2ms/90°; Image matrix= 256 × 256 x 130; voxel size=1.2mm^3	5.3
FBIRN	SCID-I/NP	No head trauma, no medical, neurological or psychiatric history, no alcohol or substance abuse in the preceding 5 years, no previous or current use of psychotropic medication, IQ>75. No history of any Axis-I psychotic disorders in 1st degree family members.	3T Siemens Tim Trio or General Electric Discovery MR750	T1-weighted SPGR; TR/TE/TI/FA=2300 ms/2.94 ms/1100 ms/9°; image matrix=256×256x160; voxel size=0.86x0.86x1.2mm^3; sagittal plane acquisition	5.1
FIDMAG	Personal interview; structured interview in part of the sample	No head trauma, no medical, neurological or psychiatric history, no lifetime alcohol or substance abuse, no previous or current use of psychotropic medication, IQ>70.	1.5 T General Electric Signa	T1-weighted MPRAGE; TR/TE/FA=2000 ms/4 ms/ 9°; image matrix=512 x 512; 180 contiguous sagittal slices; voxel size=0.56 x 0.56 x 1 mm3	5.3

GSP	Structured phone screen and study specific self-report battery and clinical screen	No head trauma, no medical, neurological or psychiatric history, no lifetime alcohol or substance abuse, no current use of psychotropic medication, normal brain anatomy following brain scan.	3T Siemens Tim Trio	T1-weighted 3D multi-echo MPRAGE; TR/TE/TI/FA =2200 ms/1.54-7 ms/ 1100/7 °; voxel size=1.2x1.2x1.2 mm	4.5
HUBIN	SCID-I	No head trauma, no medical, neurological or psychiatric history, no lifetime alcohol or substance abuse, no previous or current use of psychotropic medication, IQ>75. No history of any psychiatric disorders in 1st degree family members.	1.5 T General Electric Signa	T1-weighted SPGR; TR/TE/FA= 24 ms/6 ms/35 °; 124 coronal slices; voxel size 0.86 x 0.86 x 1.50 mm3.	5.3
HMS	Personal Interview	No head trauma, no medical, neurological or psychiatric history, no lifetime alcohol or substance abuse, no previous or current use of psychotropic medication, IQ>75. No history of any psychiatric disorders in 1st degree family members.	1.5T Siemens Magnetom Sonata	T1-weighted 3D MPRAGE; TR/TE/TI/FA=1900 ms/4.0 ms/700 ms/15°; image matrix = 256 x 256; 176 consecutive sagittal slices; voxel size=1 mm^3	5.3
IDIVAL (1) + (2)	CASH	No head trauma, no medical, neurological or psychiatric history, no lifetime alcohol or substance abuse, no previous or current use of psychotropic medication, IQ>75. No history of any psychiatric disorders in 1st degree family members.	3T Siemens Alegra, Phillips Achieva 1.5T General Electric Signa	T1-weighted SPGR; TR/TE/FA=24 ms/5 ms/ 5°; image matrix=256x192; T1-weighted SPGR; TR/TE/FA=3000 ms/3.9 ms/8°; image matrix=256x256; voxel size=1mm^3; sagittal plane acquisition	5.3
IDIVAL (3)	Personal Interview	No lifetime history of Axis I psychiatric disorders, no mild cognitive	3T Phillips Achieva	T1-weighted SPGR; TR/TE/FA=3000 ms/4.6 ms/8°; image matrix=321x312; voxel size=1mm^3; sagittal plane acquisition	5.3
IMAGEN	DAWBA questionnaire clinician interview	No head trauma, no medical, neurological or psychiatric history, no previous or current use of psychotropic medication. IQ>75	3T Siemens Verio and TimTrio, Philips Achieva, General Electric Signa Excite, and Signa HDx	T1-weighted 3D MPRAGE; TR/TE/TI/FA=2300ms/30 30ms/900ms/9°; Image matrix= 256 × 256;192 sagittal slices; voxel size=1mm^3	5.3
IMH	SCID-I/NP	No head trauma, no medical history, neurological or	3T Phillips Achieva	T1-weighted 3D MPRAGE; TR/TE/FA=	5.3

		psychiatric history, no lifetime alcohol or substance abuse, as well as no previous or current use of psychotropic medication, IQ>75. No cognitive impairment		7.2ms/ 3.8ms/8°; image matrix=256 x 256; 180 axial slices; voxel size=0.9mm^3	
IMpACT	SCID-I (and SCID-II)	No head trauma, no medical, neurological or psychiatric history, no alcohol or substance abuse in the preceding 6 months, no previous or current use of psychotropic medication, IQ>70. No history of any psychiatric disorders in 1st or 2nd degree family members.	1.5 T Siemens	T1-weighted 3D-MPRAGE; TR/TE/TI/FA =2730 ms/2.95 ms/1000 ms; 176 consecutive sagittal slices; voxel size= 1 mm^3	3.5
Indiana 1.5T	Personal Interview	No head trauma, no medical, neurological or psychiatric history, no lifetime alcohol or substance abuse, no previous or current use of psychotropic medication, IQ>75.	1.5T General Electric Signa Horizon LX	T1-weighted 3D SPGR; TR/TE/FA=25 ms/3 ms/ 45°; image matrix= 256 x 256; 124 contiguous coronal slices	5.1
Indiana 3T	Personal interview Structured phone screen	No head trauma, no medical, neurological or psychiatric history, no alcohol or substance abuse in the preceding 6 months, no previous or current use of psychotropic medication, IQ>75.	3T Siemens Skyra	T1-weighted MPRAGE; TR/TE/FA=2300 ms/2.95 ms/ 9°; image matrix=256 x 240; 176 contiguous sagittal slices	5.1
Johns Hopkins	Personal Interview	No head trauma, no medical, neurological or psychiatric history, no alcohol or substance abuse preceding 6 months, never prescribed with psychotropic medication, IQ>75. No mild cognitive impairment	1.5T General Electric Signa	T1-weighted SPGR; TR/TE/FA=35 ms/5 ms/ 45°; image matrix=256x256; 124 slices	5.3
KaSP	MINI	No head trauma, no medical, neurological or psychiatric history, no lifetime alcohol or substance abuse, no previous or current use of psychotropic medication, IQ>75. No history of any psychiatric disorders in 1st or 2nd degree family members.	3T General Electric	T1-weighted SPGR; TR/TI/FA=7.904 ms/450 ms/12 °; image matrix= 256 x 256 mm^3; 145 sagittal slices ; voxel size=0.934 x 0.934 x 1.2 mm3	5.3
Leiden	Self-report	No psychiatric or neurological disorders, no use of psychotropic medications	3T Philips Achieva	T1-weighted 3D SPGR; TR/TE = 9.76 ms/4.59 ms; image matrix=256x256; 160–180 contiguous coronal slices; voxel size=0.875x 0.875 x 1.2 mm^3	5.3
MAS	Personal interview	No head trauma, no diagnosis of dementia, schizophrenia, bipolar disorder no psychotic symptoms, no neurological	3T Philips Achieva Quasar Dual	TR/TE = 6.39 ms/2.9 ms; 190 coronal slices; voxel size = 1mm^3	5.3

		disorder, no mild cognitive impairment, IQ>75.			
MCIC	SCID, SCID-I/NP, CASH	No head trauma, no medical, neurological or psychiatric history, no lifetime alcohol or substance abuse, no previous or current use of psychotropic medication, IQ>75.	1.5T Siemens Sonata-3T Siemens Trio	T1-weighted MPRAGE sequence; TR/TE/TI/FA=2530 ms/4.76 ms/1100 ms/20°; image matrix=256×256×128 cm; voxel size=0.625 mm^3	5.3
Melbourne	SCID-I	No head trauma, no neurological or psychiatric history, no lifetime alcohol or substance abuse, no previous or current use of psychotropic medication. No history of any psychiatric disorders in 1st or 2nd degree family members.	3T GE Signa Excite	3D BRAVO sequence 140; TR/TE/FA=7900 ms/3000 ms/13°; FOV=256 mm; matrix=256 x 256	5.3
Meth-CT	SCID DSM-IV	No head trauma, no medical, neurological or psychiatric history, no lifetime alcohol or substance abuse, no previous or current use of psychotropic medication, IQ>70.	3T Siemens Allegra	T1-weighted 3D MPRAGE; TR/graded TE/FA=2530 ms/ 1.53, 3.21, 4.89, 6.57 ms/ 7°; 160 contiguous sagittal slices; voxel size=1 x 1 *x 1 mm3	5.3
MHRC	Personal interview	No head trauma, no medical history, including neurological and psychiatric history. No Family History of neurological or psychiatric disorders	3T Philips Achieva	T1-weighted TFE; TR/TE/ FA=8.2ms/3.7ms/8°; voxel size=0.83 x 0.83 x 1 mm^3	5.3
Muenster	SCID	No head trauma, no medical, neurological or psychiatric history, no lifetime alcohol or substance abuse, no previous or current use of psychotropic medication, IQ>75.	3T Phillips Intera	T1 weighted TFE: TR/TE/FA= 7.4 ms/3.4 ms/9°; image matrix = 256x204x160mm^3; voxel size=0.5mm^3; sagittal plane acquisition	5.3
NCNG	Personal interview	No head trauma, no medical, neurological or psychiatric history, no lifetime alcohol or substance abuse, no mild cognitive impairment, no previous or current use of psychotropic medication, IQ>84.	1.5T Siemens Avanto 1.5T Siemens Sonata	T1-weighted 3D MPRAGE; TR/TE/TI/FA= 2400 ms/3.61 ms/1000 ms/8°; image matrix=192x192; 160 sagittal slices; voxel size=1.25 mm^3 T1-weighted 3D MPRAGE; TR/TE/TI/FA= 2730 ms/3.43 ms/1000 ms/7°; image matrix=256x256; 128 sagittal slices; voxel size=1 mm^3	4.5
NESDA	CIDI	No lifetime history of Axis-I diagnoses, no lifetime medical or neurological morbidity including hypertension, no lifetime	3T Philips Achieva	T1-weighted 3D MPRAGE; TR/TE/FA= 9 ms/3.5 ms/8°; image matrix=256x256; 170	5.0

			SENSE-6 to 8 channel head coil	sagittal slices; voxel size=1mm³	
NeuroIMAGE	KSADS-PL	No head trauma, no mild cognitive impairment, neurological or psychiatric history, no previous or current use of psychotropic medication, IQ>75. No history of any psychiatric disorders in 1st and 2nd degree family members.	1.5 T Siemens AVANTO (Donders Centre for Cognitive Neuroimaging) 1.5 T Siemens SONATA (VU University Amsterdam)	MPRAGE 176 sagittal slices, repetition time=2,730ms, echo time=2.95ms, voxel size=1.0x1.0x1.0mm, field of view=256 mm	5.3
Neuroventure	DAWBA and BSI	No head trauma, no medical, neurological or psychiatric history, no lifetime alcohol or substance abuse, no previous or current use of psychotropic medication, IQ>75.	3T SIEMENS TrioTim	T1-weighted 3D MPRAGE; TR/TE/ FA= 2300 ms/2.96 ms/9°; image matrix= 256x256; voxel size= 1.0x1.0x1.0 mm³	5.3
NTR (1)	DISC-IV	No head trauma, no medical, neurological or psychiatric history, no lifetime alcohol or substance abuse, no mild cognitive impairment, no previous or current use of psychotropic medication, IQ>75.	1.5T Siemens Sonata	T1-weighted 3D MPRAGE; TR/TE/TI/FA=1900 ms/3.93 ms/1100 ms/ 15°; image matrix=256 x 224; 160 sagittal slices; voxel size=1 mm³	5.1
NTR (2)	MINI, BDI, STAI, STAS, YBOCS	No head trauma, no previous or current use of psychotropic medication, normal IQ.	3T Philips Intera	T1-weighted 3D MPRAGE; TR/TE/FA=9.64 ms/4.60 ms/8°; image matrix=256 x 256; 182 coronal slices; voxel size=1 x1x1.2 mm³	5.1
NTR (3)	CIDI, MADRS, BDI, STAI	No current psychiatric disorder, no current use of psychotropic medication, normal IQ.	1.5 T Siemens Sonata	T1-weighted 3D MPRAGE; TR/TE/TI/FA= 15 ms/7 ms/300 ms/8°; image matrix=256x176; 160 coronal slices; voxel size=1x1x1.5 mm³	5.1
NU	SCID	No head trauma, no medical, neurological or psychiatric history, no lifetime alcohol or substance abuse, no previous or current use of psychotropic medication, IQ>75. No history of any psychiatric disorders in 1st degree family members.	1.5T SIEMENS Vision	T1-weighted 3D MPRAGE; TR/TE/TI/FA=2200 ms/4.13 ms/766 ms/13°; voxel size =0.8mm³; axial plane acquisition.	5.3
NUIG	SCID	No head trauma, no neurological or psychiatric history, no alcohol or substance abuse preceding 6 months, no previous or current use of psychotropic medication, IQ>75. No history of any	Siemens Magnetom Symphony 1.5T	3D, T1-weighted MPRAGE 4 channel head coil, FOV 230mm, TR/TE/: 1140ms/4.38ms, matrix size 256 x 256, interpolated to 512 x 512,	5.1

Site	Interview	Inclusion/Exclusion criteria	Scanner	MRI parameters	
		psychiatric disorders in 1st degree family members.		yielding an in-plane voxel size of 0.45mm x 0.45mm^2, slice thickness 0.9mm.	
NYU	SCID-NP for DSM-IV	No head trauma, no medical history, including neurological and psychiatric history, no lifetime alcohol or substance abuse, no previous or current use of psychotropic medication. IQ>75.	3T Siemens Allegra	T1-weighted 3D MPRAGE; TR/TE/TI/FA=2530ms/3.25ms/1100ms/7°	5.3
OATS (1-4)	Personal interview	No head trauma, no current diagnosis of a psychotic disorder, no neurological disorder, no malignancy (other than skin cancer) or other severe medical comorbidity, no mild cognitive impairment, IQ>75.	1.5T Philips Gyroscan, Siemens Magnetom Avanto, Siemens Sonata; 3T Philips Achieva Quasar Dual, a	T1-weighted 3D acquisition; TR/TE/TI/FA=15370 ms/3.24 ms/780 ms/8°; 144 slices; voxel size=1 x 1 x 1.5 mm^3	5.3
OLIN	SCID I	No head trauma, no medical, neurological or psychiatric history, no alcohol or substance abuse preceding 6 months, never prescribed with psychotropic medication, IQ>75.	3T Siemens Allegra	T1-weighted 3D MPRAGE; TR/TE/TI/FA= 2300 ms/2.91 ms/900 ms/9°; image matrix= 256x240x192; 160 sagittal slices; voxel size= 1.0x1.0x1.2 mm^3	5.1
PING	Personal interview	No lifetime history of major developmental, psychiatric, or neurological disorders, brain injury, or other medical conditions that affect development. Individuals born earlier than 36 weeks of gestational age were excluded.	3T Philips Achieva 3T GE SIGNA 3T Siemens TrioTim 3T Siemens TrioTim 3T General Electric Discovery MR750	T1-weighted 3D IR-GRE; TR/TE/TI/FA= 8.1 ms/3.5 ms/640 ms/9°	5.3
QTIM	CIDI	No head trauma, no medical history, neurological and psychiatric history, no alcohol or substance abuse in the preceding 6 months, no antidepressant medication or medication affecting cognition.	4T Bruckner	T1-weighted 3D MPRAGE: TR/TE/TI/FA = 1500 ms/3.35 ms/ 700 ms/ 8°; image matrix= 256 × 256 × 256 or 256 × 256 × 240; 256 coronal slices; voxel size= 0.9 mm^3	5.1
Oxford	KSADS	No head trauma, no medical, neurological or psychiatric history, no lifetime alcohol or substance abuse, no previous or	1.5T Siemens Sonata	T1-weighted 3D MPRAGE; TR/TE =12 ms/5.6 ms; image matrix	5.3

		current use of psychotropic medication, IQ>75.		=256×240x 208 mm³; voxel size=1 mm³	
Sao Paulo (1)	SCID	No head trauma, neurological or psychiatric history, no lifetime alcohol or substance abuse.	1.5T Siemens Espree	T1-weighted 3D MPRAGE; TR/TE/TI/FA=2400 ms/3.65 ms/ 0 ms/8°; 160 contiguous sagittal slices; voxel size=1.3 x 1.3x 1.2 mm3	5.3
Sao Paulo (3)	SCID	No head trauma, neurological or psychiatric history, no lifetime alcohol or substance abuse. IQ>75	1.5T General Electric Signa	T1-weighted FSPGR ; TR/TE/TI/FA=21.7 ms/52 ms /20°; 124 axial slices; voxel size= 0.86 x 0.86 x 1.5 mm3	5.3
SCORE	BPRS	No head trauma, no medical, neurological or psychiatric history, no lifetime history of alcohol or substance abuse, no previous or current use of psychotropic medication, IQ>75. No history of any psychiatric disorders in 1st degree family members.	3T Siemens Magnetom Verio	T1-weighted 3D-MPRAGE; TR/TE/TI/FA =2000 ms/3.37 ms/1000 ms/8°; image matrix=256x256x176; 176 consecutive sagittal slices; voxel size= 1 mm³	6.0
SHIP-2	Personal Interview	No head trauma, no neurological and psychiatric history, no alcohol or substance abuse in the preceding 6 months, no previous or current use of psychotropic medication. IQ>75.	1.5T Siemens Avanto	T1-weighted 3D MPRAGE; TR/TE/ FA=1900ms/3.4ms/15°; voxel size=1mm³	5.3
SHIP-TREND	Personal Interview	No head trauma, no neurological and psychiatric history, no alcohol or substance abuse in the preceding 6 months, no previous or current use of psychotropic medication. IQ>75.	1.5T Siemens Avanto	T1-weighted 3D MPRAGE; TR/TE/ FA=1900ms/3.4ms/15°; voxel size=1 mm³	5.3
Stages-Dep	SCID-I	No head trauma, no medical, neurological or psychiatric history, no lifetime alcohol or substance abuse, no previous or current use of psychotropic medication, IQ>75. No history of any psychiatric disorders in 1st degree family members.	3T Phillips Achieva	T1-weighted 3D-MPRAGE; TR/TE/TI/FA =6.7 ms/3.2 ms/200 ms/88°; °; image matrix = 288 x 288; 170 consecutive sagittal slices; voxel size= 0.896×0.896×1.2 mm³	5.1
Stanford	SCID	No head trauma, no medical, neurological or psychiatric history, no lifetime alcohol or substance abuse, no previous or current use of psychotropic medication. no mild cognitive impairment.	1.5T General Electric Signa Excite	T1-weighted SPGR; TR/TE/TI/FA=8.3-10.3 ms/1.7-3.0 ms/300 ms/15°; image matrix= 256 x 192; 176 contiguous sagittal	5.3

				slices; voxel size=0.86x0.86x1.5 mm³; sagittal plan acquisition	
StrokeMRI	Personal interview	No head trauma, no medical, neurological or psychiatric history, no lifetime alcohol or substance abuse, no previous or current use of psychotropic medication, IQ>75.	3T General Electric Signa HDxt	T1-weighted FSPGR; TR/TE/TI/FA=7.8 s/2.956 ms/450 ms/12°; 170 slices; voxel size= 1.0x1.0x1.2 mm	5.3
Sydney	SCID	No head trauma, no medical history, neurological or psychiatric history, no alcohol or substance abuse preceding 6 months, as well as no previous or current use of psychotropic medication, IQ>75.	3T General Electric Discovery MR750	T1-weighted 3D MPRAGE; TR/TE/FA= 7264ms/ 2784ms/15°; image matrix =256 x 256 x 196; voxel size=0.9mm³	5.1
TOP	PRIME-MD	No head trauma, no organic or other psychotic disorder (ICD codes 290-299), no substance abuse in the preceding 6 months, no previous or current use of psychotropic medication, IQ>75. No history of any psychiatric disorders in 1st degree family members.	1.5T Siemens Magnetom Sonata	T1-weighted SPGR; TR/TE/TI/FA=2730 ms/3.93 ms/1000 ms/71°; voxel size = 1.33x0.94x1mm³; sagittal plane acquisition	5.3
Tuebingen	SCID I and II	No head trauma, no medical history, neurological or psychiatric history, no lifetime alcohol or substance abuse as well as no previous or current use of psychotropic medication, IQ>75. No history of any psychiatric disorders in 1st degree family members.	1.5T Siemens Avanto	T1-weighted 3D MPRAGE; TR/TE/FA= 2250ms/ 3.93ms/8°; image matrix =256 x 256; voxel size=1mm³	5.3
UMCU	CASH	No head trauma, no medical, neurological or psychiatric history, no lifetime alcohol or substance abuse, no previous or current use of psychotropic medication, IQ>75. No history of any psychiatric disorders in 1st degree family members.	1.5T Philips Intera and Achieva	T1-weighted 3D FFE; TE/TR/FA= 4.6 ms/0 ms/ 0°; 160-180 contiguous coronal slices; voxel size=1x1x1.2 mm³	5.1
UNIBA	SCID-NP	No head trauma, no medical, neurological or psychiatric history, no lifetime alcohol or substance abuse, no previous or current use of psychotropic medication, IQ>75. No history of any psychiatric disorders in 1st degree family members.	3T General Electric	T1-weighted 3D SPGR; TE/FA = min full/ 6°; image matrix= 256×256 x124	5.3
UPENN	SCID	No head trauma, no medical history, including neurological and psychiatric history, no	3T Siemens Tim Trio	T1-weighted 3D MPRAGE;	5.3

		alcohol or substance abuse preceding 6 months, no previous or current use of psychotropic medication, IQ>75. No history of any psychiatric disorders in 1st degree family members.		TR/TE/TI/FA=1810 ms/3.51 ms/1100 ms/9°; image matrix= 256 × 192;160 axial slices	
Yale	KSADS-PL	No head trauma, neurological or psychiatric history, no alcohol or substance abuse in the preceding 6 months, no previous or current use of psychotropic medication, IQ>75.	3T General Electric Signa	T1-weighted 3D MPRAGE; image matrix =256×256; voxel size=0.976 x 0.976 x 1 mm3	5.3

Abbreviations of Terms: BDI = Behavioural Descriptive Interview; BSI = Brief Symptom Inventory; CASH = Comprehensive assessment of symptoms and history; CDR = Clinical Dementia Rating; CIDI = Composite International Diagnostic Interview; DAWBA = Development and Well-Being Assessment; DISC-IV = Diagnostic Interview Schedule for Children; DSM = Diagnostic and Statistical Manual of Mental Disorders (DSM); FA=flip angle; FSPGR=fast spoiled gradient echo sequence; GRE=spoiled gradient echo sequence; ICD= International Classification of Diseases; IR= inversion recovery; KSADS-PL= Kiddie Schedule for Affective Disorders and Schizophrenia-Present and Lifetime; MADRS = Montgomery-Asberg Depression Rating Scale; MINI = Mini International Neuropsychiatric Interview; MMSE = Mini Mental State Exam; PRIME-MD = Primary Care Evaluation of Mental Disorder; SCID = Structured Clinical Interview for DSM Disorders; SCID-I/NP = SCID Non-Patient version; SPGR=spoiled gradient recalled sequence; STAI = State-Trait Anxiety Inventory; STAS = State-trait anger scale; TE=echo time; TI=inversion time; TR=repetition time; TFE=turbo field echo sequence; YBOCS = Yale-Brown Obsessive Compulsive Scale
Abbreviations of studies: ADHD-NF = Attention Deficit Hyperactivity Disorder- Neurofeedback Study; AMC = Amsterdam Medisch Centrum; Basel = University of Basel; Barcelona = University of Barcelona; Betula = Swedish longitudinal study on aging, memory, and dementia; BIG = Brain Imaging Genetics; BIL&GIN = a multimodal multidimensional database for investigating hemispheric specialization; Bonn = University of Bonn; BrainSCALE=Brain Structure and Cognition: an Adolescence Longitudinal twin study; CAMH = Centre for Addiction and Mental Health; Cardiff = Cardiff University; CEG = Cognitive-experimental and Genetic study of ADHD and Control Sibling Pairs; CIAM = Cortical Inhibition and Attentional Modulation study; CLiNG = Clinical Neuroscience Göttingen; CODE = formerly Cognitive Behavioral Analysis System of Psychotherapy (CBASP) study; Edinburgh = The University of Edinburgh; ENIGMA-HIV = Enhancing NeuroImaging Genetics through Meta-Analysis-Human Immunodeficiency Virus Working Group; ENIGMA-OCD = Enhancing NeuroImaging Genetics through Meta-Analysis- Obsessive Compulsive Disorder Working Group; FBIRN = Function Biomedical Informatics Research Network; FIDMAG = Fundación para la Investigación y Docencia Maria Angustias Giménez; GSP = Brain Genomics Superstruct Project; HMS = Homburg Multidiagnosis Study; HUBIN = Human Brain Informatics; IDIVAL = Valdecilla Biomedical Research Institute; IMAGEN = the IMAGEN Consortium; IMH=Institute of Mental Health, Singapore; IMpACT = The International Multicentre persistent ADHD Genetics Collaboration; Indiana = Indiana University School of Medicine; Johns Hopkins = Johns Hopkins University; KaSP= The Karolinska Schizophrenia Project; Leiden = Leiden University; MAS = Memory and Ageing Study; MCIC = MIND Clinical Imaging Consortium formed by the Mental Illness and Neuroscience Discovery (MIND) Institute now the Mind Research Network; Melbourne = University of Melbourne; Meth-CT = study of methamphetamine users, University of Cape Town; MHRC = Mental Health Research Center; Muenster = Muenster University; NESDA = The Netherlands Study of Depression and Anxiety; NeuroIMAGE = Dutch part of the International Multicenter ADHD Genetics (IMAGE) study; Neuroventure: the imaging part of the Co-Venture Trial funded by the Canadian Institutes of Health Research (CIHR); NCNG = Norwegian Cognitive NeuroGenetics sample; NTR = Netherlands Twin Register; NU = Northwestern University; NUIG = National University of Ireland Galway; NYU = New York University; OATS = Older Australian Twins Study; Olin = Olin Neuropsychiatric Research Center; Oxford =Oxford University; QTIM = Queensland Twin Imaging; Sao Paulo = University of Sao Paulo; SCORE = University of Basel Study; SHIP-2 and SHIP TREND = Study of Health in

Pomerania; Staged-Dep= Stages of Depression Study; Stanford = Stanford University; StrokeMRI = Stroke Magnetic Resonance Imaging; Sydney = University of Sydney; TOP = Tematisk Område Psykoser (Thematically Organized Psychosis Research); TS-EUROTRAIN = European-Wide Investigation and Training Network on the Etiology and Pathophysiology of Gilles de la Tourette Syndrome; Tuebingen = University of Tuebingen; UMCU = Universitair Medisch Centrum Utrecht; UNIBA = University of Bari Aldo Moro; UPENN=University of Pennsylvania; Yale = Yale University

2.6 Study 1 Acknowledgements, Disclosures and Funding

The full acknowledgements, disclosures and funding can be accessed via doi:

10.1002/hbm.25364

Chapter 3: Subcortical Volumes Across the Lifespan: Data from 18,605 Healthy

Individuals Aged 3-90 Years

<u>Originally published as:</u>

Dima Danai, Modabbernia Amirhossein, Papachristou Efstathios, Doucet Gaelle E, Agartz Ingrid, Aghajani Moji, Akudjedu Theophilus N et al. "Subcortical volumes across the lifespan: Data from 18,605 healthy individuals aged 3-90 years." Hum Brain Mapp. 2021 Feb 11. doi: 10.1002/hbm.25320

3.1 Study 2 Introduction

Over the last 20 years, studies using structural magnetic resonance imaging (MRI) have confirmed that brain morphometric measures change with age. In general, whole brain, global and regional gray matter volumes increase during development and decrease with aging [19,37,103-110]. However, most published studies are constrained by small sample sizes, restricted age coverage and methodological variability. These limitations introduce inconsistencies and may obscure or distort the lifespan trajectories of brain structures. To address these limitations, we formed the Lifespan Working group of the Enhancing Neuroimaging Genetics through Meta-Analysis (ENIGMA) Consortium [63,64] to perform large-scale analyses of brain morphometric data extracted from MRI images using standardized protocols and unified quality control procedures, harmonized and validated across all participating sites.

Here we focus on ventricular, striatal (caudate, putamen, nucleus accumbens), pallidal, thalamic, hippocampal and amygdala volumes. Subcortical structures are crucial for normal cognitive and emotional adaptation [111]. The striatum and pallidum (together referred to as basal ganglia) are best known for their role in action selection and movement coordination [112] but they are also involved in other aspects of cognition particularly memory, inhibitory control, reward and salience processing [113-116]. The role of the hippocampus has been most clearly defined in connection to declarative memory [117,118] while the amygdala has been historically linked to affect processing [119]. The thalamus is centrally located in the brain and acts as a key hub for the integration of motor and sensory information with higher-order functions [120,121]. The role of subcortical structures extends beyond normal cognition because changes in the volume of these regions have been reliably identified in developmental [122,123], psychiatric [49,124-126] and degenerative disorders[127].

Using data from 18,605 individuals aged 3–90 years from the ENIGMA Lifespan working group we delineated the association between age and subcortical volumes from early to late life in order to (a) identify periods of volume change or stability, (b) provide normative, age-adjusted centile curves of subcortical volumes and (c) quantify inter-individual variability in subcortical volumes which is considered a major source of inter-study differences [61,65].

3.2 Study 2 Methods

3.2.1 Study samples

The study data derive from 88 samples comprising 18,605 healthy participants, aged 3–90 years, with near equal representation of men and women (48% and 52%) (Table 1, Figure 1). At the time of scanning, participating individuals were screened to exclude the presence of mental disorders, cognitive impairment or significant medical morbidity. Details of the screening process and eligibility criteria for each research group are shown in Table S1).

Table 3.1. Characteristics of the included samples

Sample	Age, Mean, Years	Age, SD, Years	Age Range		Sample Size, N	Number of Males	Number of Females
ABIDE	17	7.8	6	56	534	439	95
ADHD NF	13	1	12	15	13	7	6
ADNI	76	5.1	60	90	150	70	80
ADNI2GO	73	6.1	56	89	133	55	78
AMC	23	3.4	17	32	92	60	32
Barcelona 1.5T	15	1.8	11	17	30	14	16
Barcelona 3T	15	2.1	11	17	44	24	20
Betula	61	12.9	25	81	234	104	130
BIG 1.5T	28	13.3	13	77	1288	628	660
BIG 3T	24	7.9	18	69	1276	540	736
BIL&GIN	27	7.8	18	57	444	217	227
Bonn	39	6.5	29	50	174	174	0
BRAINSCALE	10	1.4	9	15	270	125	145
BRCATLAS	38	15.8	18	80	153	77	76
CAMH	41	17.6	18	86	128	65	63
Cardiff	25	7.4	18	58	316	87	229
CEG	16	1.7	13	19	32	32	0
CIAM	27	5	19	40	30	16	14
CLING	25	5.3	18	58	320	131	189
CODE	40	13.3	20	64	74	31	43

COMPULS/TS							
Eurotrain	11	1	9	13	53	36	17
Dublin (1)	37	13	17	65	52	23	29
Dublin (2)	30	8.3	19	52	92	51	41
Edinburgh	24	2.9	19	31	55	35	20
ENIGMA-HIV	25	4.4	19	33	31	16	15
ENIGMA-OCD (AMC/Huyser)	14	2.6	9	17	23	9	14
ENIGMA-OCD (IDIBELL)	33	10.1	18	61	65	29	36
ENIGMA-OCD (Kyushu/Nakao)	39	12.5	22	63	40	15	25
ENIGMA-OCD (London Cohort/Mataix-Cols)	37	11.2	21	63	32	11	21
ENIGMA-OCD (van den Heuvel 1.5T)	31	7.6	21	53	48	18	30
ENIGMA-OCD (van den Heuvel 3T)	39	11.2	22	64	35	16	19
ENIGMA-OCD-3T-CONTROLS	31	10.6	19	56	27	10	17
FBIRN	37	11.2	19	60	173	123	50
FIDMAG	38	10.2	19	64	122	53	69
GSP	26	14.9	18	89	1962	860	1102
HMS	40	12.2	19	64	55	21	34
HUBIN	42	8.9	19	56	99	66	33
IDIVAL (1)	65	10.2	49	87	31	10	21
IDIVAL (3)	30	7.7	19	50	114	69	45
IDIVAL(2)	28	7.6	15	52	79	49	30
IMAGEN	14	0.4	13	16	1744	864	880
IMH	32	10	20	59	79	50	29
IMpACT-NL	37	12	19	63	134	52	82
Indiana 1.5T	60	11	37	79	41	7	34
Indiana 3T	27	18.8	6	73	197	95	102
Johns Hopkins	44	12.5	20	65	87	41	46
KaSP	27	5.7	20	43	32	15	17
Leiden	17	4.8	8	29	565	274	291
MAS	78	4.5	70	89	361	137	224
MCIC	33	12	18	60	93	63	30
Melbourne	20	3	15	26	102	54	48
METHCT	27	7.3	18	53	62	48	14
MHRC	22	2.9	16	28	52	52	0
Moods	33	9.8	18	51	310	146	164

NCNG	50	16.7	19	79	311	92	219
NESDA	40	9.8	21	56	65	22	43
NeuroIMAGE	17	3.7	8	29	376	172	204
Neuroventure	14	0.6	12	15	137	62	75
NTR (1)	15	1.4	11	18	34	11	23
NTR (2)	34	10.3	19	57	105	39	66
NTR (3)	30	5.9	20	42	29	11	18
NU	41	18.8	17	68	15	1	14
NUIG	37	11.5	18	58	89	50	39
NYU	31	8.7	19	52	51	31	20
OATS (1)	71	5.3	65	84	94	27	67
OATS (2)	68	4.4	65	81	33	13	20
OATS (3)	69	4.3	65	81	128	44	84
OATS (4)	70	4.6	65	89	95	23	72
OLIN	36	12.8	21	87	594	236	358
Oxford	16	1.4	14	19	38	18	20
PING	12	4.9	3	21	518	271	247
QTIM	23	3.4	16	30	342	112	230
Sao Paolo 1	27	5.8	17	43	69	45	24
Sao Paolo 3	30	8.1	18	50	83	44	39
SCORE	25	4.3	19	39	44	17	27
SHIP 2	55	12.3	31	84	368	206	162
SHIP TREND	50	13.9	21	81	788	439	349
StagedDep	47	8	27	59	84	20	64
Stanford	37	10.7	19	61	54	20	34
STROKEMRI	42	21.3	18	77	47	17	30
Sydney	37	21.1	12	79	147	58	89
TOP	35	9.8	18	73	296	155	141
Tuebingen	40	12.1	24	61	53	24	29
UMC Utrecht 1.5T	32	12.1	17	66	289	171	118
UMCU 3T	45	15.2	19	81	109	52	57
UNIBA	27	8.7	18	63	130	66	64
UPENN	36	13.6	16	85	185	85	100
Yale	14	2.2	10	18	23	12	11
Total	31	18.4	3	90	18605	8980	9625

N=number; SD= standard deviation

Abbreviations of studies: ABIDE=Autism Brain Imaging Data Exchange; ADNI=Alzheimer's Disease Neuroimaging Initiative; ADNI2GO=ADNI-GO and ADNI-2;ADHD-NF = Attention Deficit Hyperactivity Disorder- Neurofeedback Study; AMC = Amsterdam Medisch Centrum; Basel = University of Basel; Barcelona = University of Barcelona; Betula = Swedish longitudinal study on aging, memory, and dementia; BIG = Brain Imaging Genetics; BIL&GIN = a multimodal multidimensional database for investigating hemispheric specialization; Bonn = University of Bonn; BrainSCALE=Brain Structure and Cognition: an

Adolescence Longitudinal twin study; CAMH = Centre for Addiction and Mental Health; Cardiff = Cardiff University; CEG = Cognitive-experimental and Genetic study of ADHD and Control Sibling Pairs; CIAM = Cortical Inhibition and Attentional Modulation study; CLiNG = Clinical Neuroscience Göttingen; CODE = formerly Cognitive Behavioral Analysis System of Psychotherapy (CBASP) study; Dublin = Trinity College Dublin; Edinburgh = The University of Edinburgh; ENIGMA-HIV = Enhancing NeuroImaging Genetics through Meta-Analysis-Human Immunodeficiency Virus Working Group; ENIGMA-OCD = Enhancing NeuroImaging Genetics through Meta-Analysis- Obsessive Compulsive Disorder Working Group; FBIRN = Function Biomedical Informatics Research Network; FIDMAG = Fundación para la Investigación y Docencia Maria Angustias Giménez; GSP = Brain Genomics Superstruct Project; HMS = Homburg Multidiagnosis Study; HUBIN = Human Brain Informatics; IDIVAL = Valdecilla Biomedical Research Institute; IMAGEN = the IMAGEN Consortium; IMH=Institute of Mental Health, Singapore; IMpACT = The International Multicentre persistent ADHD Genetics Collaboration; Indiana = Indiana University School of Medicine; Johns Hopkins = Johns Hopkins University; KaSP= The Karolinska Schizophrenia Project; Leiden = Leiden University; MAS = Memory and Ageing Study; MCIC = MIND Clinical Imaging Consortium formed by the Mental Illness and Neuroscience Discovery (MIND) Institute now the Mind Research Network; Melbourne = University of Melbourne; Meth-CT = study of methamphetamine users, University of Cape Town; MHRC = Mental Health Research Center; Muenster = Muenster University; NESDA = The Netherlands Study of Depression and Anxiety; NeuroIMAGE = Dutch part of the International Multicenter ADHD Genetics (IMAGE) study; Neuroventure: the imaging part of the Co-Venture Trial funded by the Canadian Institutes of Health Research (CIHR); NCNG = Norwegian Cognitive NeuroGenetics sample; NTR = Netherlands Twin Register; NU = Northwestern University; NUIG = National University of Ireland Galway; NYU = New York University; OATS = Older Australian Twins Study; Olin = Olin Neuropsychiatric Research Center; Oxford =Oxford University; QTIM = Queensland Twin Imaging; Sao Paulo = University of Sao Paulo; SCORE = University of Basel Study; SHIP-2 and SHIP TREND = Study of Health in Pomerania; Staged-Dep= Stages of Depression Study; Stanford = Stanford University; StrokeMRI = Stroke Magnetic Resonance Imaging; Sydney = University of Sydney; TOP = Tematisk Område Psykoser (Thematically Organized Psychosis Research); TS-EUROTRAIN = European-Wide Investigation and Training Network on the Etiology and Pathophysiology of Gilles de la Tourette Syndrome; Tuebingen = University of Tuebingen; UMCU = Universitair Medisch Centrum Utrecht; UNIBA = University of Bari Aldo Moro; UPENN=University of Pennsylvania; Yale = Yale University

---

3.2.2 Neuroimaging

Detailed information on scanner vendor, magnet strength and acquisition parameters for each sample are presented in Table S1. For each sample, the intracranial volume (ICV) and the volume of the basal ganglia (caudate, putamen, pallidum, nucleus accumbens), thalamus, hippocampus, amygdala and lateral ventricles were extracted using FreeSurfer (http://surfer.nmr.mgh.harvard.edu) from high-resolution T_1-weighted MRI brain scans [66,67]. Prior to data pooling, images were visually inspected at each site to exclude participants whose scans were improperly segmented. After merging the samples, only individuals with complete data were included outliers were identified and excluded using Mahalanobis distances. All analyses described below were repeated for ICV-unadjusted volumetric measures which yielded identical results and are only presented as a separate supplement.

Approximately 20% of the samples had a multi-scanner design. During data harmonization the scanner was modeled as batch effect instead of site. In each site, the intracranial volume (Figure S1) was used to adjust the subcortical volumes via a formula based on the analysis of the covariance approach: "adjusted volume = raw volume $- b \times$ (ICV $-$ mean ICV)", where b is the slope of regression of a region of interest volume on ICV [37]. The values of the subcortical volumes were then harmonized between sites using the ComBat method in R [70,71,128]. Originally developed to adjust for batch effect in genetic studies, ComBat uses an empirical Bayes to adjust for inter-site variability in the data, while preserving variability related to the variables of interest.

3.2.3 Fractional polynomial regression analyses

The effect of age on each ICV- and site-adjusted subcortical volume was modeled using high order fractional polynomial regression [68,69] in each hemisphere. Because the effect of the scanner was adjusted using ComBat, we only included sex as a covariate in the regression models. Fractional polynomial regression is currently considered the most advantageous modeling strategy for continuous variables [129] as it allows testing for a wider range of trajectory shapes than conventional lower-order polynomials (e.g., linear or quadratic) and for multiple turning points [68,130]. For each subcortical structure, the best model was obtained by comparing competing models of up to three power combinations. The powers used to identify the best fitting model were −2, −1, −0.5, 0.5, 1, 2, 3 and the natural logarithm (ln) function. The optimal model describing the association between age and each of the volumes was selected as the lowest degree model based on the partial F-test (if linear) or the likelihood-ratio test. To avoid over-fitting at ages with more data points, we used the stricter .01 level of significance as the cut-off for each respective likelihood-ratio tests, rather than adding powers, until the .05 level was reached. For ease of interpretation, we centered the volume of each structure so that the intercept of a fractional polynomial was represented as the effect at zero for sex. Fractional polynomial regression models were fitted using Stata/IC software v.13.1 (Stata Corp., College Station, TX). Standard errors were also adjusted for the effect of site in the FP regression.

We conducted two supplemental analyses: (a) we specified additional FP models separately for males and females and, (b) we calculated Pearson's correlation coefficient between subcortical volumes and age in the early (6–29 years), middle (30–59 years), and late-life (60–90 years) age-group. The results of these analyses have been included in the supplemental material.

3.2.4 Inter-individual variability

Inter-individual variability was assessed using two complimentary approaches. First, for each subcortical structure we compared the early (6–29 years), middle (30–59 years) and late-life (60–90 years) age-groups in terms of their mean inter-individual variability; these groups were defined following conventional notions regarding periods of development, midlife and aging. The variance of each structure in each age-group was calculated as

$$\ln\left(\frac{\sum\sqrt{e_i^2}}{n_t}\right)$$

where e represents the residual variance of each individual (i) around the nonlinear best fitting regression line, and n the number of observations in each age-group (t). The residuals (e_i) were normally distributed suggesting good fit of the model without having over- or under-fitted the data. Upon calculating the square root of the squared residuals, we used the natural logarithm to account for the positive skewness of the new distribution. Then the mean inter-individual variability between early (6–29 years), middle (30–59 years) and late-life (60–90 years) age-groups was compared using

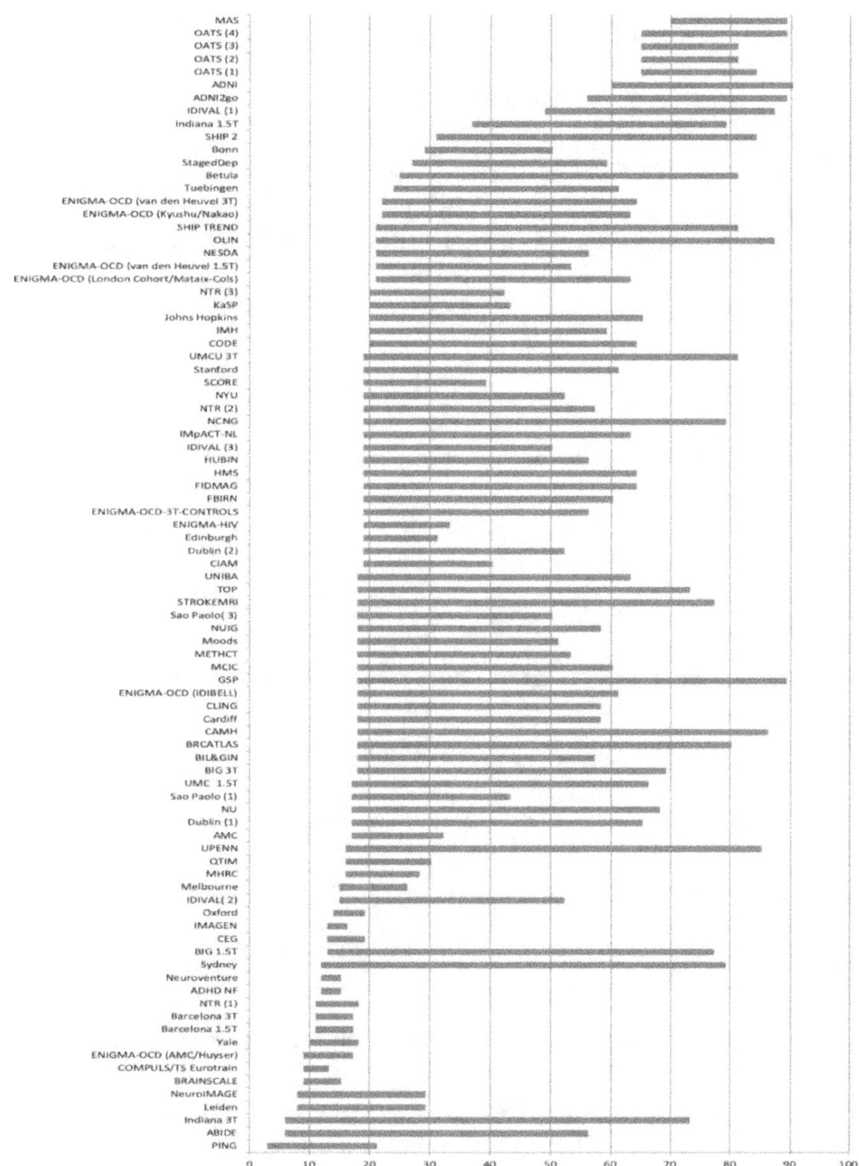

Figure 3.1. Age range for each sample
Abbreviations are explained in Table 1 and further details of each sample are provided
in the supplemental material.

between-groups omnibus tests for the residual variance around the identified best-fitting nonlinear fractional polynomial model of each structure. We conducted 16 tests (one for each structure) and accordingly the critical alpha value was set at 0.003 following Bonferroni correction for multiple comparisons.

The second approach entailed the quantification of the mean individual variability of each subcortical structure through a meta-analysis of the *SD* of the adjusted volumes according to the method proposed by Senior et al [72].

3.2.5 Centile curves

Reference curves for each structure by sex and hemisphere were produced from ICV- and site-adjusted volumes as normalized growth centiles using the parametric Lambda (λ), Mu (μ), Sigma (σ) (LMS) method [131] implemented using the Generalized Additive Models for Location, Scale and Shape (GAMLSS) version 5.2-0 in R (http://cran.r-project.org/web/packages/gamlss/index.html) [73,74]. LMS allows for the estimation of the distribution at each covariate value after a suitable transformation and is summarized using three smoothing parameters, the Box-Cox power λ, the mean μ and the coefficient of variation σ. GAMLSS uses an iterative maximum (penalized) likelihood estimation method to estimate λ, μ and σ as well as distribution dependent smoothing parameters and provides optimal values for effective degrees of freedom (edf) for every parameter [75]. This procedure minimizes the Generalized Akaike Information Criterion (GAIC) goodness of fit index; smaller GAIC values indicate better fit of the model to the data. GAMLSS is a flexible way to derive normalized centile curves as it allows each curve to have its own number of edf while overcoming biased estimates resulting from skewed

data.

3.3 Study 2 Results

3.3.1 Fractional polynomial regression analyses

The volume of the caudate, putamen, globus pallidus and nucleus accumbens

peaked early during the first decade of life and showed a linear decline immediately

thereafter (Figure 2, Figures S2-S4). The association between age and the volumes of the

thalamus, hippocampus and amygdala formed a flattened, inverted U-curve (Figure 3,

Figures S5 and S6). Specifically, the volumes of these structures were largest during the

first 2–3 decades of life, remained largely stable until the sixth decade and declined

gradually thereafter (Table S2). The volume of the lateral ventricles increased steadily

with age bilaterally (Figure S7). The smallest proportion of variance explained by age and

its FP derivatives was noted in the right amygdala (7%) and the largest in the lateral

ventricles bilaterally (38%) (Table S2). Striatal volumes correlated negatively with age

throughout the lifespan with the largest coefficients observed in the middle-life age-

group ($r = -0.39$ to -0.20) and the lowest ($|r| < 0.05$) in the late-life age-group, particularly

in the caudate. The volumes of the thalamus, the hippocampus and the amygdala showed

small positive correlations with age ($r \approx 0.16$) in the early-life age-group. In the middle-

life age-group, the correlation between age and subcortical volumes became negative ($r =$

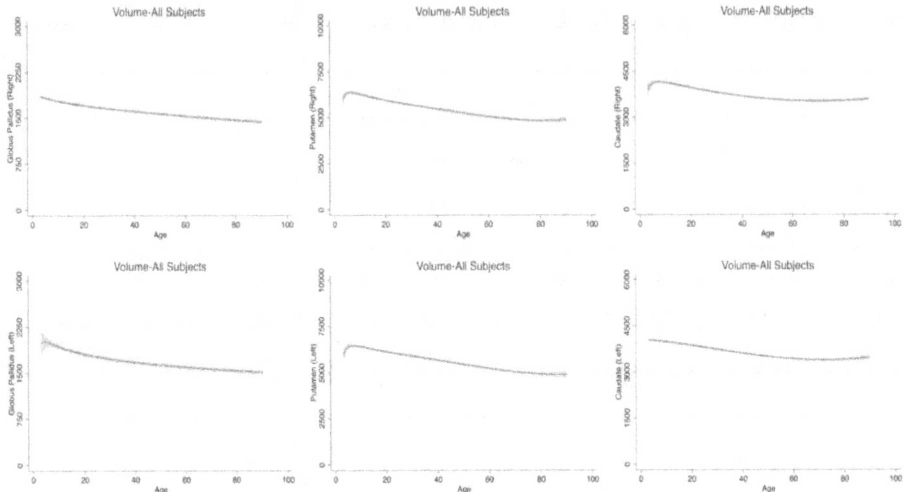

Figure 3.2. Fractional Polynomial Plots for the Volume of the Right (Top) and Left (Bottom) Globus Pallidus (Left), Putamen (Middle) and Caudate (Right)

Fractional Polynomial plots of adjusted basal ganglia volumes (mm^3) against age (years) with a fitted regression line (solid line) and 95% confidence intervals (shaded area).

–0.30 to –0.27) for the thalamus but remained largely unchanged for the amygdala and the hippocampus. In the late-life age-group, the largest negative correlation coefficients between age and volume were observed for the hippocampus bilaterally (r = –0.44 to –0.39). The correlation between age and lateral ventricular volumes bilaterally increased throughout the lifespan from r = 0.19 to 0.20 in early-life age-group to r = 0.40 to 0.45 in the late-life age-group (Table S3). No effect of sex was noted for any pattern of correlation between subcortical volumes and age in any age-group.

3.3.2 Inter-individual variability

For each structure, the mean inter-individual variability in volume in each age-group is shown in Table S5. Inter-individual variance was significantly higher for the

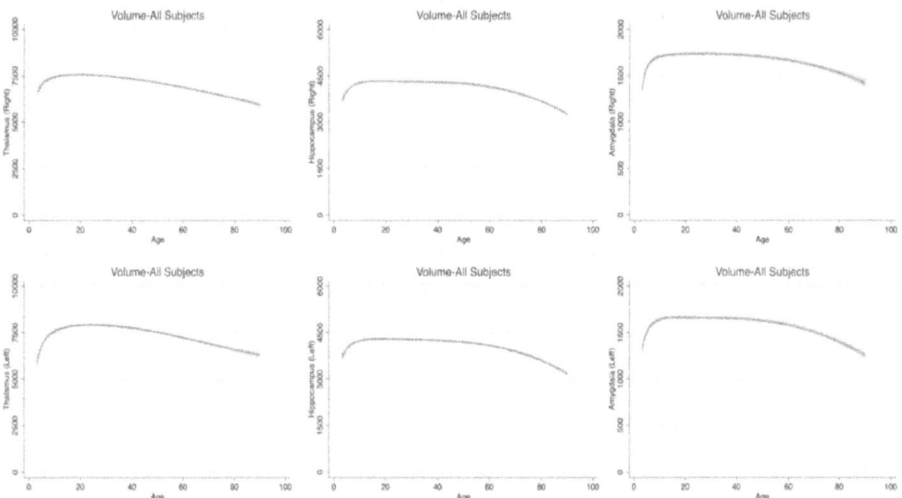

Figure 3.3. Fractional Polynomial Plots for the Volume of the Right (Top) and Left
(Bottom) Thalamus (Left), Hippocampus (Middle) and Amygdala (Right)
Fractional Polynomial plots of adjusted thalamus, hippocampal and amygdala volumes
(mm^3) against age (years) with a fitted regression line (solid line) and 95% confidence
intervals (shaded area).

hippocampus, thalamus amygdala and lateral ventricles bilaterally in the late-life age-group compared to both the early- and middle-life group. These findings were recapitulated when data were analyzed using a meta-analytic approach (Figure S8).

Normative Centile Curves: Centile normative values for each subcortical structure stratified by sex and hemisphere are shown in Figure 4 and Table S6-S8

3.4 Study 2 Discussion

We analyzed subcortical volumes from 18,605 healthy individuals from multiple cross-sectional cohorts to infer age-related trajectories between the ages of 3 and 90 years.

Our lifespan perspective and our large sample size complement and enrich previous age-related findings in subcortical volumes.

We found three distinct patterns of association between age and subcortical

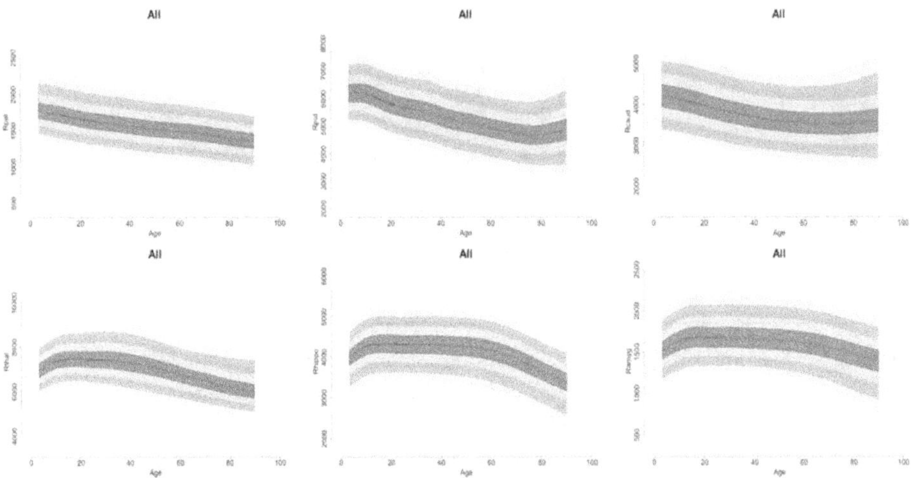

Figure 3.4. Normative Centile Curves for the Volume of the Right Globus Pallidus (Top Left), Putamen (Top Center), Caudate (Top Left), Thalamus (Bottom Left), Hippocampus (Bottom Center) and Amygdala (Bottom Right)
Normative centile curves of adjusted right basal ganglia, thalamus, hippocampal and amygdala volumes (mm^3) against age (years). From center outward, the shades show 50% , 25% and 75%, 10% and 90%, 5 and 95%, 2.5 % and 97.5%, and 1% and 99%.

volumes. The volume of the lateral ventricles increased monotonically with age. Striatal

and pallidal volumes peaked in childhood and declined thereafter. The volumes of the

thalamus, hippocampus and amygdala peaked later and showed a prolonged period of

stability lasting until the sixth decade of life, before they also started to decline. These

findings are in line with those of Pompino et al[107], who also used harmonized multi-site

MRI data from 10,323 individuals aged 3–96 years, and those reported by Douaud et al.

[132] who analyzed volumetric data from 484 healthy participants aged 8 to 85 years.

Notably, both studies reported similarity in the age-related changes of the thalamus, hippocampus and the amygdala. Our results also underscore the significantly steeper negative association between subcortical volumes and age from the sixth decade of life onwards. This effect seemed relatively more pronounced for the hippocampus, compared to the other subcortical regions, as observed in other studies [61,107,133]

The trajectories of subcortical volumes are shaped by genetic and nongenetic exposures, biological or otherwise [134-136]. Our findings of higher inter-individual variability with age in the volumes of the thalamus, hippocampus and amygdala suggest that these structures may be more susceptible to person-specific exposures, or late-acting genes, particularly from the sixth decade onwards.

The unique strengths of this study are the availability of age-overlapping cross-sectional data from healthy individuals, lifespan coverage and the use of standardized protocols for volumetric data extraction across all samples. Study participants in each site were screened to ensure mental and physical wellbeing at the time of scanning using procedures considered as standard in designating study participants as healthy controls. Although health is not a permanent attribute, it is extremely unlikely given the size of the sample that the results could have been systematically biased by incipient disease

A similar longitudinal design would be near infeasible in terms of recruitment and retention both of participants and investigators. Although multisite studies have to account for differences in scanner type and acquisition, lengthy longitudinal designs encounter similar issues due to inevitable changes in scanner type and strength and acquisition parameters over time. In this study, the use of age-overlapping samples from multiple different countries has the theoretical advantage of diminishing systematic biases reflecting cohort and period effects [137,138] that are likely to operate in single site studies.

In medicine, biological measures from each individual are typically categorized as normal or otherwise in reference to a population derived normative range. This approach is yet to be applied to neuroimaging data, despite the widespread use of structural MRI for clinical purposes and the obvious benefit of a reference range from the early identification of deviance [65,107]. Alzheimer's disease provides an informative example as the degree of baseline reduction in medial temporal regions, and particularly the hippocampus, is one of the most significant predictors of conversion from mild cognitive impairment to Alzheimer's disease [127]. The data presented here demonstrate the power of international collaborations within ENIGMA for analyzing large-scale datasets that could eventually lead to normative range for brain volumes for well-defined reference populations. The centile curves presented here are a first step in developing normative reference values for neuroimaging phenotypes and further work is required in establishing measurement error and functional significance (see Supplement). These curves are not meant to be used clinically or to provide valid percentile measures for a single individual.

In conclusion, we used existing cross-sectional data to infer age-related trajectories of regional subcortical volumes. The size and age-coverage of the analysis sample has the potential to disambiguate uncertainties regarding developmental and aging changes in subcortical volumes while the normative centile values could be further developed and evaluated.

3.5 Study 2 Supplemental Material

Due to very large volume of the supplemental files, important tables and figures are presented below and the rest are available only online. The full supplemental material for this study can be accessed online through the following link: https://onlinelibrary.wiley.com/action/downloadSupplement?doi=10.1002%2Fhbm.2532 0&file=hbm25320-sup-0001-AppendixS1.zip

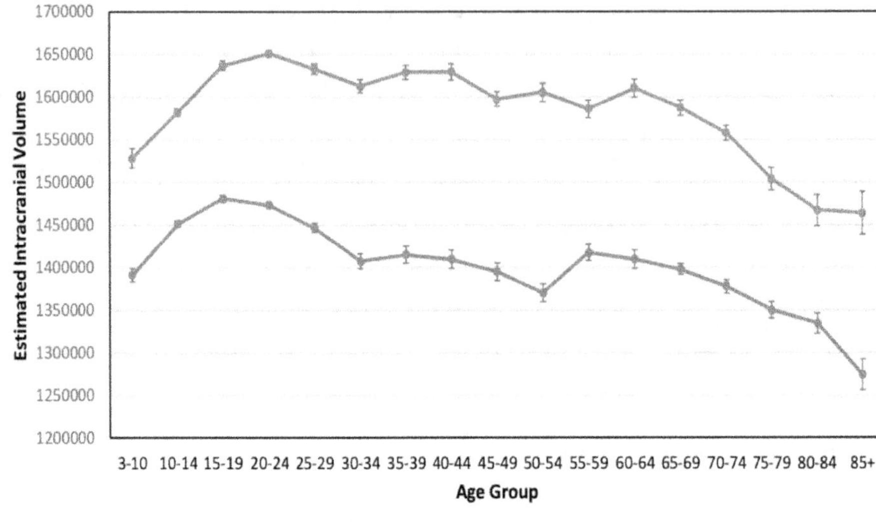

Figure S1. Intracranial volume (ICV) by Sex and Age (mean, standard error)

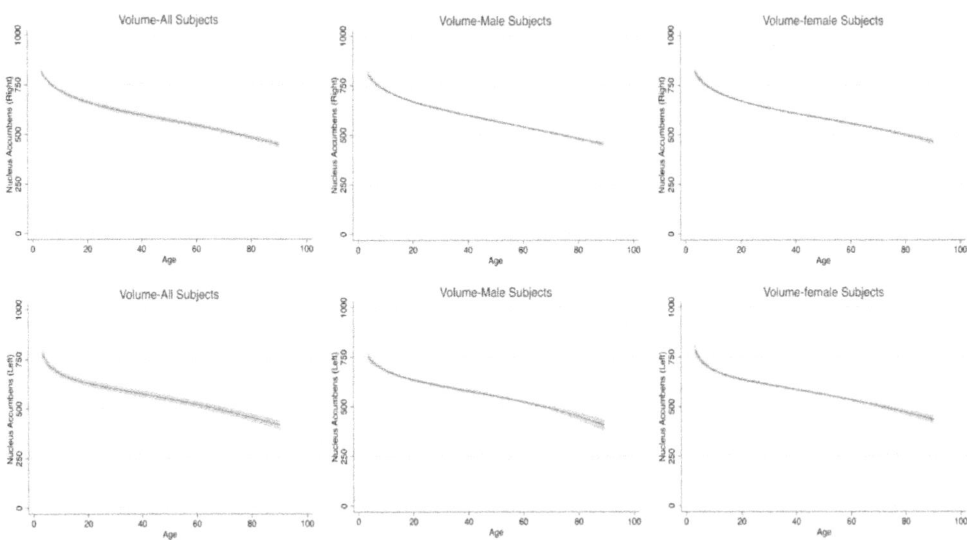

Figure S6. Age-related Trajectories in the right (Top) and Left (bottom) Nucleus Accumbens for All (Left), Male (Middle), and Female (Right) subjects.

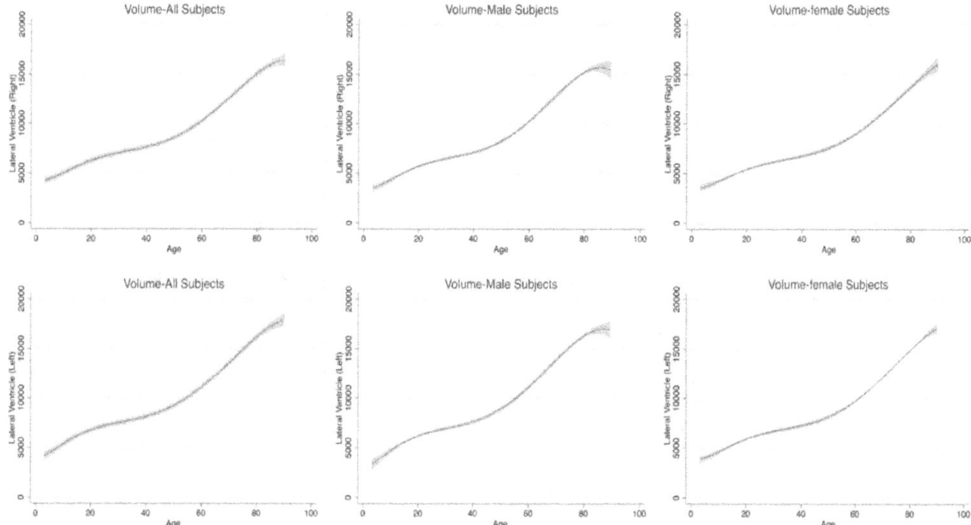

Figure S7. Age-related Trajectories in the right (Top) and Left (bottom) Lateral Ventricles for All (Left), Male (Middle), and Female (Right) subjects.

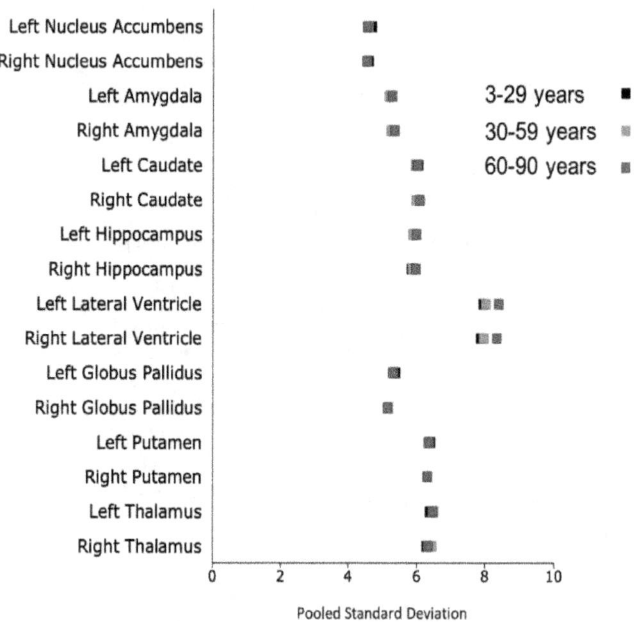

Figure S8. Meta-analysis of Pooled Standard Deviation

69

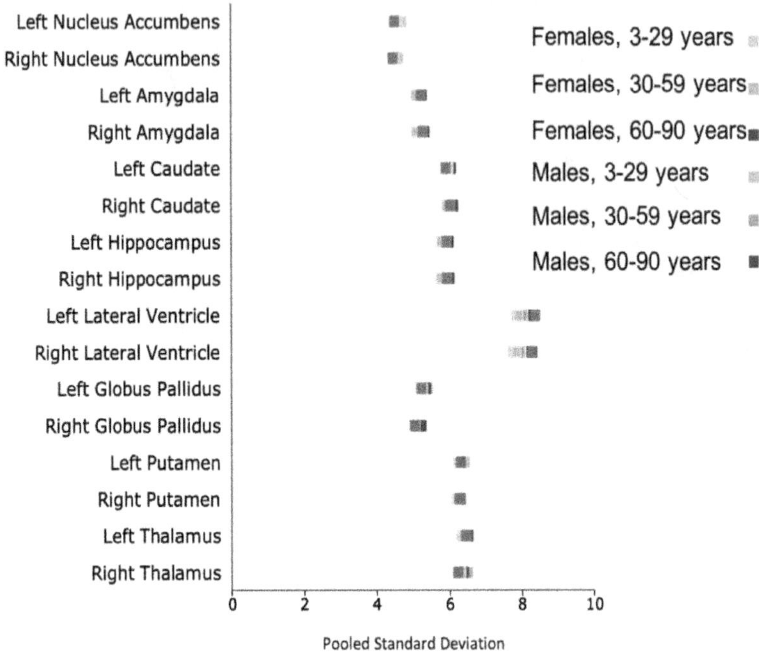

Figure S9. Meta-analysis of Pooled Standard Deviation Stratified by Sex

Table S1. Screening Process and Eligibility Criteria, Scanner, Image Acquisition Parameters and Image Segmentation Software

Sample	Screening Process	Eligibility Criteria	Magnet strength / Scanner Vendor	Acquisition parameters	Freesurfer version
ABIDE	Autism Diagnostic Observation Schedule/ Autism Diagnostic Interview-R	No head trauma, no medical, neurological or psychiatric history, no previous or current use of psychotropic medication, IQ>75.	3T Siemens Magnet om Tim Trio, 3T Siemens Magnet om Veiro, 3T Philips Achieva, 3T Siemens	T1-weighted MPRAGE; TR/TE/TI/ FA= 1590 ms /2.7 ms /800 ms/ 10 °; image matrix=256x256x176; voxel size=1mm³; sagittal plane acquisition; T1-weighted MPRAGE; TR/TE/TI/FA= 1870 ms /2.48 ms/1100 ms/8 °; image matrix==350x263x350; voxel size=1mm³; sagittal plane acquisition; T1-weighted MPRAGE; TR/TE/TI /FA= 8 ms/3.7 ms/843 ms/8 °; image	5.0

			MAGNETOM Allegra, 3T General Electric, Philips 3 T, 3T GE Signa, Philips 3 T Interna,	matrix=256x200x200; voxel size=1mm³; coronal plane acquisition; T1-weighted MPRAGE; TR/TE/TI/FA= 1800 ms/3.06 ms/900 ms/9 °; image matrix=256x240x160; voxel size=1mm3; sagittal plane acquisition; T1-weighted MPRAGE; TR/TE/TI/ FA = 2530 ms /3.25 ms /1100 ms/ 7 °; image matrix=256x256x171; voxel size=1.3x1x1.3mm³; sagittal plane acquisition; T1-weighted MPRAGE; TR/TE/TI /FA= 2000 ms /230 ms/600 ms/8 °; sagittal plane acquisition; T1-weighted MPRAGE; TR/TE/ FA= 8.4 ms /1.8 ms/15 °; image matrix=256x132x256; voxel size=0.86x1.5x0.86 mm³ T1-weighted MPRAGE; TR/TE/FA= 9.6 ms/3.6 ms/8 °; image matrix=250x218x250; voxel size=0.98x0.98x1.2 mm³; coronal plane acquisition	
ADNI	Personal Interview	MMSE scores of 24-30, CDR=0, no current depressive symptoms, no mild cognitive impairment	1.5T Various Vendors	T1-weighted 3D MPRAGE: Representative imaging parameters: TR/TE/TI/FA=2400 ms/3.5 ms/1000 m/8 °; image matrix=192x192; 160 sagittal slices; voxel size= 0.94x0.94x1.2 mm³	5.1
ADNI2GO	Personal Interview	Within normative range in the Wechsler Memory Scale; MMSE score of 24-30; CDR =0; Memory Box score = 0; no significant impairment in cognitive functions or activities of daily living.	3T Various Vendors	T1-weighted 3D MPRAGE: Representative imaging parameters :TR/TE/FA=400 ms/60s/11 °; image matrix=256 x 256; sagittal plane acquisition	5.1
ADHD-NF	KSADS	No head trauma, no neurological and psychiatric history, no lifetime alcohol or substance abuse, no previous or current use of psychotropic medication, IQ>75.	3T Siemens Tim Trio	T1-weighted 3D MPRAGE; TR/TE/TI/FA=2300ms/3030ms/900 ms/9°; Image matrix= 256 × 256; 192 sagittal slices; voxel size=1mm³	5.3
AMC	Personal Interview	No head trauma, no medical, neurological or psychiatric history, no lifetime alcohol or substance abuse, no previous or current use of psychotropic medication, IQ>75. No history of any psychiatric disorders in 1st degree family members.	3T Philips Intera	T1-weighted 3D MPRAGE; TE range= 3.5-4.6ms, TR range= 9-9.663ms, FA=	5.1

Barcelona 1.5T	KSADS	No head trauma, no medical, neurological or psychiatric history, no lifetime alcohol or substance abuse, no previous or current use of psychotropic medication, IQ>75. No history of any psychiatric disorders in 1st degree family members.	1.5 T General Electric Signa	T1-weighted; image matrix = 256 x 256; 128 slices; voxel size 1 x 1 x 1 mm^3.	5.3
Barcelona 3T	KSADS	No head trauma, no medical, neurological or psychiatric history, no lifetime alcohol or substance abuse, no previous or current use of psychotropic medication, IQ>75. No history of any psychiatric disorders in 1st degree family members.	3 T Siemens MAGNETOM TIM Trio	T1-weighted; image matrix = 256 x 256; 240 slices; voxel size 1 x 1 x 1 mm^3.	5.3
Betula	Personal Interview	No head trauma, no medical, neurological or psychiatric history, no lifetime alcohol or substance abuse, no previous or current use of psychotropic medication.	3T General Electric Discovery MR750	T1-weighted MPRAGE; TR/TE/TI/FA=8.1240 ms/3.2000 ms/450ms/ 12°; image matrix = 256x256	5.3
BIG	Questionnaire for psychiatric history	No head trauma, no medical, neurological or psychiatric history, no lifetime alcohol or substance abuse, no previous or current use of psychotropic medication, IQ>70. No history of any psychiatric disorders in 1st or 2nd degree family members.	1,5 T Siemens Sonata and Avanto and 3 T Siemens Trio, TimTrio and Skyra	T1-weighted 3D MPRAGE; TR/TE/TI/sagittal slices = 1940-2730 ms/850-110 ms/2.92-4.58 ms; 176-192 sagittal slices; voxel size= 1.0x1.0x1.0 mm^3	5.3
BIL&GIN	Personal Interview	No head trauma, no current neurological or psychiatric disorders, no current use of psychotropic medication, IQ>70.	3T Phillips ACHIEVA	T1 - weighted 3D; TR/TE/TI/FA=20 ms/4.6 ms/800ms/ 10°; turbo field echo factor = 65; sense factor = 2; matrix size = 256x256x180mm 3 ; voxel size= 1.0x1.0x1.0 mm^3	5.3
Bonn	Personal interview	No head trauma, no medical, neurological or psychiatric history, no previous or current use of psychotropic medication.	3T Siemens Trio	TR/TE/FA= 1570-1660ms/2.75-3.42ms/8-9°	NA
BrainSCALE	Personal interview	No head trauma, no medical, neurological or psychiatric history, no lifetime alcohol or substance abuse, no previous or current use of psychotropic medication.	1.5T Phillips Achieva	T1-weighted 3D SPGR; TR/TE/FA= 30 ms/4.6 ms/30°; image matrix=256x256; 160–180 contiguous coronal slices; voxel size=1 x 1 x 1.2 mm^3	5.1
BRCATLAS	Telephone interview	No head trauma, no medical, neurological or psychiatric	3T GE Signa	T1-weighted 3D; TR/TE/TI/FA= 6.9 ms/2.8 ms/650 ms/8°; Image matrix	

Site	Diagnostic	Inclusion/Exclusion criteria	Scanner	Imaging parameters	Version
CAMH	SCID	history, no lifetime alcohol or substance abuse, no mild cognitive impairment, no previous or current use of psychotropic medication, IQ>75. No head trauma, no neurological or psychiatric history, no alcohol or substance abuse preceding 6 months, no previous or current use of psychotropic medication, IQ>75. No history of any psychotic disorders in 1st degree family members.	1.5 T GE (echospeed)	124 Axial inversion recovery–prepared spoiled gradient recall images, 1.5-mm-thick slice acquisition TE/TR/TI/FA=5.3ms/12.3ms/300.0 ms/20°.	5.3
Cardiff	MINI	No head trauma, no medical history, including neurological and psychiatric history, no alcohol or substance abuse in the preceding 6 months, no previous or current use of psychotropic medication.	3T General Electric Signa	T1-weighted 3D FSPGR; TR/TE/TI/FA=7.9ms/3.0ms/450ms/20°; Image matrix= 256 × 192 x 172; voxel size=1mm^3	5.3
CEG	Teacher and parent Conners'	No head trauma, no medical history, including neurological and psychiatric history, no alcohol or substance abuse in the preceding 6 months, no previous or current use of psychotropic medication. IQ>75	3T General Electric Signa	T1-weighted 3D SPGR; TR/TE/FA=2000ms/30ms/90°; Image matrix= 128 × 128; 43 slices	5.3
CIAM	SCID	No head trauma or psychiatric history, no previous or current use of psychotropic medication, IQ>75.	3T Siemens Allegra	T1-weighted 3D MPRAGE; TR/TE/TI/FA= 2530 ms/1.53, 3.21, 4.89, 6.57/2.91 ms/ ms/7°; image matrix= 256x256; 128 sagittal slices; voxel size= 1.3x1.0x1.3 mm^3	5.3
CLiNG	Personal Interview	No head trauma, no medical, neurological or psychiatric history, no lifetime alcohol or substance abuse, no previous or current use of psychotropic medication, IQ>75. No history of any psychiatric disorders in 1st degree family members.	3T Siemens Tim Trio	T1-weighted 3D MPRAGE; TR/TE/TI/FA=2250 ms/3.26 ms/900 ms/9°; image matrix = 256 x 256; 192 sagittal slices; voxel size= 1 mm^3	5.3
CODE	SCID	No head trauma, no medical, neurological or psychiatric history, no lifetime alcohol or substance abuse, no previous or current use of psychotropic medication, IQ>75. No history of any psychiatric disorders in 1st degree family members.	3T Siemens Trio (4 CODE sites); 3T Philips Achieva (1 CODE site)	Siemens: T1 mprage, 1mm isotropic voxels, 12 channel head coil, TR=1900ms, TE=2.52ms, 170/192 slices. Philips: T1 3D-TFE, 1mm isotropic voxels, 8 channel head coil, TR=8.3ms, TE=3.8ms, 170 slices	5.3

COMPULS /TS EUROTRA IN	KSADS	No head trauma, no medical, neurological or psychiatric history, no alcohol or substance abuse preceding 6 months, no previous or current use of psychotropic medication, IQ>75. No history of any psychiatric disorders in 1st or 2nd degree family members.	3T Siemens Tim Trio and Prisma	T1-weighted 3D MPRAGE; TR/TE/FA=2300 ms/2.98 ms/9°; image matrix = 256 x 256; 176 sagittal slices; voxel size= 1x1x1.2 mm^3	5.3
Dublin (1)	SCID-I	No head trauma, no medical history, including neurological and psychiatric history, no alcohol or substance abuse preceding 6 months, as well as no previous or current use of psychotropic medication, IQ>75.	1.5T Siemens	T1-weighted MPRAGE; TR/TE= 11.6 ms/4.9 ms; image matrix=512 x 512	5.3
Dublin (2)	SCID-I	No head trauma, no medical history, including neurological and psychiatric history, no alcohol or substance abuse preceding 6 months, as well as no previous or current use of psychotropic medication, IQ>75.	3T Phillips Intera and Achieva	T1-weighted 3D FFE; TE/TR/FA=3.8 ms/8.4 ms/88°; image matrix= 256 x 256; 180 slices; voxel size=0.9 mm^3	5.3
Edinburgh	SCID-NP	No head trauma, no medical, neurological or psychiatric history, no previous or current use of psychotropic medication, IQ>75. No history of any psychiatric disorders in 1st and 2nd degree family members.	1.5T Siemens Magnet om Essenza 1.5T General Electric Signa	T1-weighted MPRAGE; TR/TE/TI/FA =10 ms/4 ms/200 ms/8°; 128 contiguous coronal slices; voxel size=1.25 x 1.25 x 1.20 mm T1-weighted MPRAGE; TR/TE/TI/FA =10 ms/4 ms/500 ms/8°; image matrix = 192 x 192; 180 coronal slices; voxel size=1.25 x 1.25 x 1.2 mm3	5.3
ENIGMA-HIV	MINI	No head trauma, no medical, neurological or psychiatric history, no alcohol or substance abuse preceding 6 months, no previous or current use of psychotropic medication, IQ>75. No mild cognitive impairment	3T Siemens Allegra	T1-weighted MPRAGE; TR/TE/TI/FA=2400 ms/2.38 ms/1000 ms/ 8°; 162 slices; voxel size= 1 mm^3	5.1
ENIGMA-OCD (3T OCD control)	MINI-Plus	No head trauma, no medical, neurological or psychiatric history, no lifetime alcohol or substance abuse, no previous or current use of psychotropic medication, IQ>75. No cognitive impairment	3T Siemens Allegra	T1-weighted 3D MPRAGE; TR/TE/TI/FA=2300 ms/3.93 ms/ 1100 ms/12°; image matrix =256×240; 160 contiguous sagittal slices; voxel size=1.3 x 1 x 1 mm^3	5.3

ENIGMA-OCD (van den Heuvel 1.5T)	SCID-I	No medical or psychiatric history	1.5T Siemens Sonata	T1-weighted 3D MPRAGE; TR/TE/TI/FA=2700 ms/4 ms/ 950 ms/8°; image matrix =256×192; 160 slices; voxel size= 1 mm^3	5.3
ENIGMA-OCD (van den Heuvel 3T)	SCID-I	No medical or psychiatric history	3T General Electric Signa	T1-weighted 3D MPRAGE; image matrix =256×256; 172 slices; voxel size= 1x0.977x0.977 mm^3	5.3
ENIGMA-OCD (Huyser)	Personal Interview	No head trauma, no medical, neurological or psychiatric history, no lifetime alcohol or substance abuse, no previous or current use of psychotropic medication, IQ>75.	3T Phillips Intera	T1-weighted 3D MPRAGE; TR/TE/ FA=9.69 ms/4.60 ms/8°; image matrix =256×256; 182 slices; voxel size=1 x 1 x 1.2 mm^3	5.3
ENIGMA-OCD (Mataix-Cols)	SCID	No head trauma, no neurological or psychiatric history, no lifetime alcohol or substance abuse, no previous or current use of psychotropic medication, IQ>75.	1.5T General Electric Signa	T1-weighted 3D SPGR; TR/TE/FA= 14.8 ms/ 1.7 ms/ 20°; image matrix= 256 x 256 x 124; voxel size: 0.94 x 0.94 x 1.50 mm	5.3
ENIGMA-OCD (Nakao)	Personal Interview	No head trauma, no neurological or psychiatric history, no lifetime alcohol or substance abuse.	3T Phillips Achieva	T1-weighted 3D TFE; TR/TE/TI/FA=8.2 ms/3.8ms/1026 ms/8°; image matrix =240×240; 190 slices; voxel size=1 mm^3	5.3
ENIGMA-OCD (IDIBELL)	SCID-I/NP	No head trauma, no medical, neurological or psychiatric history, no alcohol or substance abuse in the preceding 6 months, no previous or current use of psychotropic medication, IQ>70. No history of any psychiatric disorders in 1st or 2nd degree family members	1.5 T General Electric Signa	T1-weighted 3D FSPGR; TR/TE/ FA=11.8ms/4.2ms/90°; Image matrix= 256 × 256 x 130; voxel size=1.2mm^3	5.3
FBIRN	SCID-I/NP	No head trauma, no medical, neurological or psychiatric history, no alcohol or substance abuse in the preceding 5 years, no previous or current use of psychotropic medication, IQ>75. No history of any Axis-I psychotic disorders in 1st degree family members.	3T Siemens Tim Trio or General Electric Discovery MR750	T1-weighted SPGR; TR/TE/TI/FA=2300 ms/2.94 ms/1100 ms/9°; image matrix=256×256x160; voxel size=0.86x0.86x1.2mm^3; sagittal plane acquisition	5.1
FIDMAG	Personal interview; structured interview in part of	No head trauma, no medical, neurological or psychiatric history, no lifetime alcohol or substance abuse, no previous	1.5 T General Electric Signa	T1-weighted MPRAGE; TR/TE/FA=2000 ms/4 ms/ 9°; image matrix=512 x 512; 180 contiguous sagittal slices; voxel size=0.56 x 0.56 x 1 mm3	5.3

	the sample	or current use of psychotropic medication, IQ>70.			
GSP	Structured phone screen and study specific self-report battery and clinical screen	No head trauma, no medical, neurological or psychiatric history, no lifetime alcohol or substance abuse, no current use of psychotropic medication, and normal brain anatomy following brain scan.	3T Siemens Tim Trio	T1-weighted 3D multi-echo MPRAGE; TR/TE/TI/FA =2200 ms/1.54-7 ms/ 1100/7 °; voxel size=1.2x1.2x1.2 mm	4.5
HUBIN	SCID-I	No head trauma, no medical, neurological or psychiatric history, no lifetime alcohol or substance abuse, no previous or current use of psychotropic medication, IQ>75. No history of any psychiatric disorders in 1st degree family members.	1.5 T General Electric Signa	T1-weighted SPGR; TR/TE/FA= 24 ms/6 ms/35 °; 124 coronal slices; voxel size 0.86 x 0.86 x 1.50 mm3.	5.3
HMS	Personal Interview	No head trauma, no medical, neurological or psychiatric history, no lifetime alcohol or substance abuse, no previous or current use of psychotropic medication, IQ>75. No history of any psychiatric disorders in 1st degree family members.	1.5T Siemens Magnetom Sonata	T1-weighted 3D MPRAGE; TR/TE/TI/FA=1900 ms/4.0 ms/700 ms/15°; image matrix = 256 x 256; 176 consecutive sagittal slices; voxel size=1 mm^3	5.3
IDIVAL (1) + (2)	CASH	No head trauma, no medical, neurological or psychiatric history, no lifetime alcohol or substance abuse, no previous or current use of psychotropic medication, IQ>75. No history of any psychiatric disorders in 1st degree family members.	3T Siemens Alegra, Phillips Achieva 1.5T General Electric Signa	T1-weighted SPGR; TR/TE/FA=24 ms/5 ms/ 5°; image matrix=256x192; T1-weighted SPGR; TR/TE/FA=3000 ms/3.9 ms/8°; image matrix=256x256; voxel size=1mm^3; sagittal plane acquisition	5.3
IDIVAL (3)	Personal Interview	No lifetime history of Axis I psychiatric disorders, no mild cognitive	3T Phillips Achieva	T1-weighted SPGR; TR/TE/FA=3000 ms/4.6 ms/8°; image matrix=321x312; voxel size=1mm^3; sagittal plane acquisition	5.3
IMAGEN	DAWBA questionnaire clinician interview	No head trauma, no medical, neurological or psychiatric history, no previous or current use of psychotropic medication. IQ>75	3T Siemens Verio and TimTrio , Philips Achieva , General Electric	T1-weighted 3D MPRAGE; TR/TE/TI/FA=2300ms/3030ms/900 ms/9°; Image matrix= 256 × 256;192 sagittal slices; voxel size=1mm^3	5.3

Site					
			Signa Excite, and Signa HDx		
IMH	SCID-I/NP	No head trauma, no medical history, neurological or psychiatric history, no lifetime alcohol or substance abuse, as well as no previous or current use of psychotropic medication, IQ>75. No cognitive impairment	3T Phillips Achieva	T1-weighted 3D MPRAGE; TR/TE/FA= 7.2ms/ 3.8ms/8°; image matrix=256 x 256; 180 axial slices; voxel size=0.9mm^3	5.3
IMpACT-NL	SCID-I (and SCID-II)	No head trauma, no medical, neurological or psychiatric history, no alcohol or substance abuse in the preceding 6 months, no previous or current use of psychotropic medication, IQ>70. No history of any psychiatric disorders in 1st or 2nd degree family members.	1.5 T Siemens	T1-weighted 3D-MPRAGE; TR/TE/TI/FA =2730 ms/2.95 ms/1000 ms; 176 consecutive sagittal slices; voxel size= 1 mm^3	3.5
Indiana 1.5T	Personal Interview	No head trauma, no medical, neurological or psychiatric history, no lifetime alcohol or substance abuse, no previous or current use of psychotropic medication, IQ>75.	1.5T General Electric Signa Horizon LX	T1-weighted 3D SPGR; TR/TE/FA=25 ms/3 ms/ 45°; image matrix= 256 x 256; 124 contiguous coronal slices	5.1
Indiana 3T	Personal interview Structured phone screen	No head trauma, no medical, neurological or psychiatric history, no alcohol or substance abuse in the preceding 6 months, no previous or current use of psychotropic medication, IQ>75.	3T Siemens Skyra	T1-weighted MPRAGE; TR/TE/FA=2300 ms/2.95 ms/ 9°; image matrix=256 x 240; 176 contiguous sagittal slices	5.1
Johns Hopkins	Personal Interview	No head trauma, no medical, neurological or psychiatric history, no alcohol or substance abuse preceding 6 months, never prescribed with psychotropic medication, IQ>75. No mild cognitive impairment	1.5T General Electric Signa	T1-weighted SPGR; TR/TE/FA=35 ms/5 ms/ 45°; image matrix=256x256; 124 slices	5.3
KaSP	MINI	No head trauma, no medical, neurological or psychiatric history, no lifetime alcohol or substance abuse, no previous or current use of psychotropic medication, IQ>75. No history of any psychiatric disorders in	3T General Electric	T1-weighted SPGR; TR/TI/FA=7.904 ms/450 ms/12°; image matrix= 256 x 256 mm^3; 145 sagittal slices ; voxel size=0.934 x 0.934 x 1.2 mm3	5.3

		1st or 2nd degree family members.			
Leiden	Self-report	No psychiatric or neurological disorders, no use of psychotropic medications	3T Philips Achieva	T1-weighted 3D SPGR; TR/TE = 9.76 ms/4.59 ms; image matrix=256x256; 160–180 contiguous coronal slices; voxel size=0.875x 0.875 x 1.2 mm^3	5.3
MAS	Personal interview	No head trauma, no diagnosis of dementia, schizophrenia, bipolar disorder no psychotic symptoms, no neurological disorder, no mild cognitive impairment, IQ>75.	3T Philips Achieva Quasar Dual	TR/TE = 6.39 ms/2.9 ms; 190 coronal slices; voxel size = 1mm^3	5.3
MCIC	SCID, SCID-I/NP, CASH	No head trauma, no medical, neurological or psychiatric history, no lifetime alcohol or substance abuse, no previous or current use of psychotropic medication, IQ>75.	1.5T Siemens Sonata-3T Siemens Trio	T1-weighted MPRAGE sequence; TR/TE/TI/FA=2530 ms/4.76 ms/1100 ms/20°; image matrix=256×256×128 cm; voxel size=0.625 mm^3	5.3
Melbourne	SCID-I	No head trauma, no neurological or psychiatric history, no lifetime alcohol or substance abuse, no previous or current use of psychotropic medication. No history of any psychiatric disorders in 1st or 2nd degree family members.	3T GE Signa Excite	3D BRAVO sequence 140; TR/TE/FA=7900 ms/3000 ms/13°; FOV=256 mm; matrix=256 x 256	5.3
Meth-CT	SCID DSM-IV	No head trauma, no medical, neurological or psychiatric history, no lifetime alcohol or substance abuse, no previous or current use of psychotropic medication, IQ>70.	3T Siemens Allegra	T1-weighted 3D MPRAGE; TR/graded TE/FA=2530 ms/ 1.53, 3.21, 4.89, 6.57 ms/ 7°; 160 contiguous sagittal slices; voxel size=1 x 1 *x 1 mm3	5.3
MHRC	Personal interview	No head trauma, no medical history, including neurological and psychiatric history. No Family History of neurological or psychiatric disorders	3T Philips Achieva	T1-weighted TFE; TR/TE/ FA=8.2ms/3.7ms/8°; voxel size=0.83 x 0.83 x 1 mm^3	5.3
Moods	Personal Interview	No head trauma, no medical, neurological or psychiatric history, no lifetime alcohol or substance abuse, no previous or current use of psychotropic medication, IQ>75. No history of any psychiatric disorders in 1st degree family members.	3T Siemens Trio	T1-weighted 3D MPRAGE; TR/TE/FA=1570 ms/2.75 ms/15o; image matrix =256x256; voxel size = 1mm3	5.1
NCNG	Personal interview	No head trauma, no medical, neurological or psychiatric history, no lifetime alcohol or substance abuse, no mild	1.5T Siemens Avanto	T1-weighted 3D MPRAGE; TR/TE/TI/FA= 2400 ms/3.61 ms/1000 ms/8°; image	4.5

		cognitive impairment, no previous or current use of psychotropic medication, IQ>84.	1.5T Siemens Sonata	matrix=192x192; 160 sagittal slices; voxel size=1.25 mm³ T1-weighted 3D MPRAGE; TR/TE/TI/FA= 2730 ms/3.43 ms/1000 ms/7°; image matrix=256x256; 128 sagittal slices; voxel size=1 mm³	
NESDA	CIDI	No lifetime history of Axis-I diagnoses, no lifetime medical or neurological morbidity including hypertension, no lifetime substance dependence, no substance abuse in the preceding year, no medication use.	3T Philips Achieva SENSE-6 to 8 channel head coil	T1-weighted 3D MPRAGE; TR/TE/FA= 9 ms/3.5 ms/8°; image matrix=256x256; 170 sagittal slices; voxel size=1mm³	5.0
NeuroIMAGE	KSADS-PL	No head trauma, no mild cognitive impairment, neurological or psychiatric history, no previous or current use of psychotropic medication, IQ>75. No history of any psychiatric disorders in 1st and 2nd degree family members.	1.5 T Siemens AVANTO (Donders Centre for Cognitive Neuroimaging)	MPRAGE 176 sagittal slices, repetition time=2,730ms, echo time=2.95ms, voxel size=1.0x1.0x1.0mm, field of view=256 mm	5.3
Neuroventure	DAWBA and BSI	No head trauma, no medical, neurological or psychiatric history, no lifetime alcohol or substance abuse, no previous or current use of psychotropic medication, IQ>75.	1.5 T Siemens SONATA (VU University Amsterdam) 3T SIEMENS TrioTim	T1-weighted 3D MPRAGE; TR/TE/ FA= 2300 ms/2.96 ms/9°; image matrix= 256x256; voxel size= 1.0x1.0x1.0 mm³	5.3
NTR (1)	DISC-IV	No head trauma, no medical, neurological or psychiatric history, no lifetime alcohol or substance abuse, no mild cognitive impairment, no previous or current use of psychotropic medication, IQ>75.	1.5T Siemens Sonata	T1-weighted 3D MPRAGE; TR/TE/TI/FA=1900 ms/3.93 ms/1100 ms/ 15°; image matrix=256 x 224; 160 sagittal slices; voxel size=1 mm³	5.1
NTR (2)	MINI, BDI, STAI,	No head trauma, no previous or current use of psychotropic medication, normal IQ.	3T Philips Intera	T1-weighted 3D MPRAGE; TR/TE/FA=9.64 ms/4.60 ms/8°; image matrix=256 x 256; 182 coronal slices; voxel size=1 x1x1.2 mm³	5.1

	STAS, YBOCS				
NTR (3)	CIDI, MADRS, BDI, STAI	No current psychiatric disorder, no current use of psychotropic medication, normal IQ.	1.5 T Siemens Sonata	T1-weighted 3D MPRAGE; TR/TE/TI/FA= 15 ms/7 ms/300 ms/8°; image matrix=256x176; 160 coronal slices; voxel size=1x1x1.5 mm^3	5.1
NU	SCID	No head trauma, no medical, neurological or psychiatric history, no lifetime alcohol or substance abuse, no previous or current use of psychotropic medication, IQ>75. No history of any psychiatric disorders in 1st degree family members.	1.5T SIEME NS Vision	T1-weighted 3D MPRAGE; TR/TE/TI/FA=2200 ms/4.13 ms/766 ms/13°; voxel size =0.8mm^3; axial plane acquisition.	5.3
NUIG	SCID	No head trauma, no neurological or psychiatric history, no alcohol or substance abuse preceding 6 months, no previous or current use of psychotropic medication, IQ>75. No history of any psychiatric disorders in 1st degree family members.	Siemens Magnet om Sympho ny 1.5T	3D, T1-weighted MPRAGE 4 channel head coil, FOV 230mm, TR/TE/: 1140ms/4.38ms, matrix size 256 x 256, interpolated to 512 x 512, yielding an in-plane voxel size of 0.45mm x 0.45mm^2, slice thickness 0.9mm.	5.1
NYU	SCID-NP for DSM-IV	No head trauma, no medical history, including neurological and psychiatric history, no lifetime alcohol or substance abuse, no previous or current use of psychotropic medication. IQ>75.	3T Siemens Allegra	T1-weighted 3D MPRAGE; TR/TE/TI/FA=2530ms/3.25ms/1100ms/7°	5.3
OATS (1-4)	Personal interview	No head trauma, no current diagnosis of a psychotic disorder, no neurological disorder, no malignancy (other than skin cancer) or other severe medical comorbidity, no mild cognitive impairment, IQ>75.	1.5T Philips Gyrosca n, Siemens Magnet om Avanto, Siemens Sonata; 3T Philips Achieva Quasar Dual, a	T1-weighted 3D acquisition; TR/TE/TI/FA=15370 ms/3.24 ms/780 ms/8°; 144 slices; voxel size=1 x 1 x 1.5 mm^3	5.3
OLIN	SCID I	No head trauma, no medical, neurological or psychiatric history, no alcohol or substance abuse preceding 6 months, never prescribed with psychotropic medication, IQ>75.	3T Siemens Allegra	T1-weighted 3D MPRAGE; TR/TE/TI/FA= 2300 ms/2.91 ms/900 ms/9°; image matrix= 256x240x192; 160 sagittal slices; voxel size= 1.0x1.0x1.2 mm^3	5.1

PING	Personal interview	No lifetime history of major developmental, psychiatric, or neurological disorders, brain injury, or other medical conditions that affect development. Individuals born earlier than 36 weeks of gestational age were excluded.	3T Philips Achieva 3T GE SIGNA 3T Siemens TrioTim 3T Siemens TrioTim 3T General Electric Discovery MR750	T1-weighted 3D IR-GRE; TR/TE/TI/FA= 8.1 ms/3.5 ms/640 ms/9°	5.3
QTIM	CIDI	No head trauma, no medical history, neurological and psychiatric history, no alcohol or substance abuse in the preceding 6 months, no antidepressant medication or medication affecting cognition.	4T Bruckner	T1-weighted 3D MPRAGE: TR/TE/TI/FA = 1500 ms/3.35 ms/ 700 ms/ 8°; image matrix= 256 × 256 × 256 or 256 × 256 × 240; 256 coronal slices; voxel size= 0.9 mm^3	5.1
Oxford	KSADS	No head trauma, no medical, neurological or psychiatric history, no lifetime alcohol or substance abuse, no previous or current use of psychotropic medication, IQ>75.	1.5T Siemens Sonata	T1-weighted 3D MPRAGE; TR/TE =12 ms/5.6 ms; image matrix =256×240x 208 mm^3; voxel size=1 mm^3	5.3
Sao Paulo (1)	SCID	No head trauma, neurological or psychiatric history, no lifetime alcohol or substance abuse.	1.5T Siemens Espree	T1-weighted 3D MPRAGE; TR/TE/TI/FA=2400 ms/3.65 ms/ 0 ms/8°; 160 contiguous sagittal slices; voxel size=1.3 x 1.3x 1.2 mm3	5.3
Sao Paulo (3)	SCID	No head trauma, neurological or psychiatric history, no lifetime alcohol or substance abuse. IQ>75	1.5T General Electric Signa	T1-weighted FSPGR ; TR/TE/TI/FA=21.7 ms/52 ms /20°; 124 axial slices; voxel size= 0.86 x 0.86 x 1.5 mm3	5.3
SCORE	BPRS	No head trauma, no medical, neurological or psychiatric history, no lifetime history of alcohol or substance abuse, no previous or current use of psychotropic medication, IQ>75. No history of any psychiatric disorders in 1st degree family members.	3T Siemens Magnetom Verio	T1-weighted 3D-MPRAGE; TR/TE/TI/FA =2000 ms/3.37 ms/1000 ms/8°; image matrix=256x256x176; 176 consecutive sagittal slices; voxel size= 1 mm^3	6.0
SHIP-2	Personal Interview	No head trauma, no neurological and psychiatric history, no alcohol or	1.5T Siemens Avanto	T1-weighted 3D MPRAGE; TR/TE/ FA=1900ms/3.4ms/15°; voxel size=1mm^3	5.3

		substance abuse in the preceding 6 months, no previous or current use of psychotropic medication. IQ>75.			
SHIP-TREND	Personal Interview	No head trauma, no neurological and psychiatric history, no alcohol or substance abuse in the preceding 6 months, no previous or current use of psychotropic medication. IQ>75.	1.5T Siemens Avanto	T1-weighted 3D MPRAGE; TR/TE/ FA=1900ms/3.4ms/15°; voxel size=1 mm³	5.3
Staged-Dep	SCID-I	No head trauma, no medical, neurological or psychiatric history, no lifetime alcohol or substance abuse, no previous or current use of psychotropic medication, IQ>75. No history of any psychiatric disorders in 1st degree family members.	3T Phillips Achieva	T1-weighted 3D-MPRAGE; TR/TE/TI/FA =6.7 ms/3.2 ms/200 ms/88°; °; image matrix = 288 x 288; 170 consecutive sagittal slices; voxel size= 0.896×0.896×1.2 mm³	5.1
Stanford	SCID	No head trauma, no medical, neurological or psychiatric history, no lifetime alcohol or substance abuse, no previous or current use of psychotropic medication. no mild cognitive impairment.	1.5T General Electric Signa Excite	T1-weighted SPGR; TR/TE/TI/FA=8.3-10.3 ms/1.7-3.0 ms/300 ms/15°; image matrix= 256 x 192; 176 contiguous sagittal slices; voxel size=0.86x0.86x1.5 mm³; sagittal plan acquisition	5.3
StrokeMRI	Personal interview	No head trauma, no medical, neurological or psychiatric history, no lifetime alcohol or substance abuse, no previous or current use of psychotropic medication, IQ>75.	3T General Electric Signa HDxt	T1-weighted FSPGR; TR/TE/TI/FA=7.8 s/2.956 ms/450 ms/12°; 170 slices; voxel size= 1.0x1.0x1.2 mm	5.3
Sydney	SCID	No head trauma, no medical history, neurological or psychiatric history, no alcohol or substance abuse preceding 6 months, as well as no previous or current use of psychotropic medication, IQ>75.	3T General Electric Discovery MR750	T1-weighted 3D MPRAGE; TR/TE/FA= 7264ms/ 2784ms/15°; image matrix =256 x 256 x 196; voxel size=0.9mm³	5.1
TOP	PRIME-MD	No head trauma, no organic or other psychotic disorder (ICD codes 290-299), no substance abuse in the preceding 6 months, no previous or current use of psychotropic medication, IQ>75. No history of any psychiatric disorders in 1st degree family members.	1.5T Siemens Magnetom Sonata	T1-weighted SPGR; TR/TE/TI/FA=2730 ms/3.93 ms/1000 ms/71°; voxel size = 1.33x0.94x1mm³; sagittal plane acquisition	5.3

Tuebingen	SCID I and II	No head trauma, no medical history, neurological or psychiatric history, no lifetime alcohol or substance abuse as well as no previous or current use of psychotropic medication, IQ>75. No history of any psychiatric disorders in 1st degree family members.	1.5T Siemens Avanto	T1-weighted 3D MPRAGE; TR/TE/FA= 2250ms/ 3.93ms/8°; image matrix =256 x 256; voxel size=1mm³	5.3
UMCU	CASH	No head trauma, no medical, neurological or psychiatric history, no lifetime alcohol or substance abuse, no previous or current use of psychotropic medication, IQ>75. No history of any psychiatric disorders in 1st degree family members.	1.5T Philips Intera and Achieva	T1-weighted 3D FFE; TE/TR/FA= 4.6 ms/0 ms/ 0°; 160-180 contiguous coronal slices; voxel size=1x1x1.2 mm³	5.1
UNIBA	SCID-NP	No head trauma, no medical, neurological or psychiatric history, no lifetime alcohol or substance abuse, no previous or current use of psychotropic medication, IQ>75. No history of any psychiatric disorders in 1st degree family members.	3T General Electric	T1-weighted 3D SPGR; TE/FA = min full/ 6°; image matrix= 256×256 x124	5.3
UPENN	SCID	No head trauma, no medical history, including neurological and psychiatric history, no alcohol or substance abuse preceding 6 months, no previous or current use of psychotropic medication, IQ>75. No history of any psychiatric disorders in 1st degree family members.	3T Siemens Tim Trio	T1-weighted 3D MPRAGE; TR/TE/TI/FA=1810 ms/3.51 ms/1100 ms/9°; image matrix= 256 × 192;160 axial slices	5.3
Yale	KSADS-PL	No head trauma, neurological or psychiatric history, no alcohol or substance abuse in the preceding 6 months, no previous or current use of psychotropic medication, IQ>75.	3T General Electric Signa	T1-weighted 3D MPRAGE; image matrix =256×256; voxel size=0.976 x 0.976 x 1 mm3	5.3

Abbreviations of Terms: BDI = Behavioural Descriptive Interview; BSI = Brief Symptom Inventory; CASH = Comprehensive assessment of symptoms and history; CDR = Clinical Dementia Rating; CIDI = Composite International Diagnostic Interview; DAWBA = Development and Well-Being Assessment; DISC-IV = Diagnostic Interview Schedule for Children; DSM = Diagnostic and Statistical Manual of Mental Disorders (DSM); FA=flip angle; FSPGR=fast spoiled gradient echo sequence; GRE=spoiled gradient echo sequence; ICD= International Classification of Diseases; IR= inversion recovery; KSADS-PL= Kiddie Schedule for Affective Disorders and Schizophrenia-Present and Lifetime; MADRS = Montgomery-Asberg Depression Rating Scale; MINI = Mini International Neuropsychiatric Interview; MMSE = Mini Mental State Exam; PRIME-MD = Primary Care Evaluation of Mental Disorder; SCID = Structured Clinical Interview for DSM Disorders; SCID-I/NP = SCID Non-Patient version; SPGR=spoiled gradient recalled sequence; STAI = State-Trait Anxiety Inventory; STAS = State-trait anger scale; TE=echo time; TI=inversion time; TR=repetition time; TFE=turbo field echo sequence; YBOCS = Yale-Brown Obsessive Compulsive Scale Abbreviations of studies: ABIDE=Autism Brain Imaging Data Exchange; ADNI=Alzheimer's Disease Neuroimaging Initiative; ADNI2GO=ADNI-GO and ADNI-2;ADHD-NF = Attention Deficit Hyperactivity Disorder-Neurofeedback Study; AMC = Amsterdam Medisch Centrum; Basel = University of Basel; Barcelona = University of Barcelona; Betula = Swedish longitudinal study on aging, memory, and dementia; BIG = Brain Imaging Genetics; BIL&GIN = a multimodal multidimensional database for investigating hemispheric specialization; Bonn = University of Bonn; BrainSCALE=Brain Structure and Cognition: an Adolescence Longitudinal twin study; CAMH = Centre for Addiction and Mental Health; Cardiff = Cardiff University; CEG = Cognitive-experimental and Genetic study of ADHD and Control Sibling Pairs; CIAM = Cortical Inhibition and Attentional Modulation study; CLiNG = Clinical Neuroscience Göttingen; CODE = formerly Cognitive Behavioral Analysis System of Psychotherapy (CBASP) study; Dublin = Trinity College Dublin; Edinburgh = The University of Edinburgh; ENIGMA-HIV = Enhancing NeuroImaging Genetics through Meta-Analysis-Human Immunodeficiency Virus Working Group; ENIGMA-OCD = Enhancing NeuroImaging Genetics through Meta-Analysis- Obsessive Compulsive Disorder Working Group; FBIRN = Function Biomedical Informatics Research Network; FIDMAG = Fundación para la Investigación y Docencia Maria Angustias Giménez; GSP = Brain Genomics Superstruct Project; HMS = Homburg Multidiagnosis Study; HUBIN = Human Brain Informatics; IDIVAL = Valdecilla Biomedical Research Institute; IMAGEN = the IMAGEN Consortium; IMH=Institute of Mental Health, Singapore; IMpACT = The International Multicentre persistent ADHD Genetics Collaboration; Indiana = Indiana University School of Medicine; Johns Hopkins = Johns Hopkins University; KaSP= The Karolinska Schizophrenia Project; Leiden = Leiden University; MAS = Memory and Ageing Study; MCIC = MIND Clinical Imaging Consortium formed by the Mental Illness and Neuroscience Discovery (MIND) Institute now the Mind Research Network; Melbourne = University of Melbourne; Meth-CT = study of methamphetamine users, University of Cape Town; MHRC = Mental Health Research Center; Muenster = Muenster University; NESDA = The Netherlands Study of Depression and Anxiety; NeuroIMAGE = Dutch part of the International Multicenter ADHD Genetics (IMAGE) study; Neuroventure: the imaging part of the Co-Venture Trial funded by the Canadian Institutes of Health Research (CIHR); NCNG = Norwegian Cognitive NeuroGenetics sample; NTR = Netherlands Twin Register; NU = Northwestern University; NUIG = National University of Ireland Galway; NYU = New York University; OATS = Older Australian Twins Study; Olin = Olin Neuropsychiatric Research Center; Oxford =Oxford University; QTIM = Queensland Twin Imaging; Sao Paulo = University of Sao Paulo; SCORE = University of Basel Study; SHIP-2 and SHIP TREND = Study of Health in Pomerania; Staged-Dep= Stages of Depression Study; Stanford = Stanford University; StrokeMRI = Stroke Magnetic Resonance Imaging; Sydney = University of Sydney; TOP = Tematisk Område Psykoser (Thematically Organized Psychosis Research); TS-EUROTRAIN = European-Wide Investigation and Training Network on the Etiology and Pathophysiology of Gilles de la Tourette Syndrome; Tuebingen = University of Tuebingen; UMCU = Universitair Medisch Centrum Utrecht; UNIBA = University of Bari Aldo Moro; UPENN=University of Pennsylvania; Yale = Yale University

3.6 Study 2 Acknowledgements, Disclosures and Funding

The full acknowledgements, disclosures and funding can be accessed via doi:

10.1002/hbm.25320

Chapter 4: Linked Patterns of Biological and Environmental Covariation with Brain Structure in Adolescence: a Population-Based Longitudinal Study

Originally published as:

Amirhossein Modabbernia, Abraham Reichenberg, Alex Ing, Dominik A Moser, Gaelle E Doucet, Eric Artiges, Tobias Banaschewski, et al. Mol Psychiatry. 2020 May 22;10.1038/s41380-020-0757-x. doi: 10.1038/s41380-020-0757-x

4.1 Study 3 Introduction

Adolescence is a critical period for brain maturation leading to adult-levels of emotional self-regulation and cognitive control [8,9,139]. At the same time, this period of brain reorganization is also associated with increased vulnerability to psychopathology [4,140,141]; the incidence of psychiatric disorders increases exponentially after the age of 10 years with 75% of cases being diagnosed by age 24 years[142,143]. Factors that influence adolescent brain development are therefore critical in forming the foundation for both positive and negative adult functional outcomes [4,140,141].

A substantial body of literature has documented the typical brain structural changes observed during adolescence; cortical thickness shows a largely monotonic decrease [144,145], cortical surface area expands and subcortical structures show individual variation in terms of expansion and contraction [108,146]. These developmental trajectories are shaped by the dynamic interplay between biologically programmed functions ("nature") and social and physical exposures ("nurture"). Age and biological sex are implicitly associated with biologically programmed functions as normal adolescent development follows predictable timelines and is sexually dimorphic [145,147,148]. Key social and physical exposures known to influence adolescent brain organization include perinatal events [149,150], parental socioeconomic status [151,152], parenting style [153] and social adversity [154]. Additionally, associations with brain structure have been noted for personal characteristics such as cognitive abilities [38,155] personality and behavioural traits [156-158].

Despite progress, the current literature is limited in several respects. Prior studies have typically examined either a single or very few of the non-imaging factors that can influence adolescent brain development; this narrow focus ignores the fact that many of these factors may be correlated. Notably, multivariate analyses in adults have identified a "positive-negative" axis of co-variation between brain phenotypes and multiple individual attributes; those that are considered positive (e.g., higher cognitive abilities) generally show positive covariation with imaging phenotypes while the opposite is the case for attributes or indicators considered negative (e.g. substance use) [159-161]. Such multivariate analyses of developmental data require large longitudinal samples, which have typically not been available in studies in youth [157,162-164]. Therefore, the appropriate modelling of the multiple factors associated with adolescent brain development remains a key unmet priority [165].

To address these challenges, the current study applied sparse canonical correlation analysis (sCCA) [166], a machine learning technique, to define associations between adolescent brain structural development with a broad array of factors indicating biological programming (age and sex), personal attributes, and social and environmental influences. We capitalised on the rich database of the IMAGEN Study (https://imagen-europe.com/) which provided high-quality brain structural imaging data collected from a population-derived cohort of more than 2000 youth. In addition, the dataset includes non-imaging variables that describe participants' demographic, anthropometric, lifestyle, psychometric and behavioural features as well as their family function and social circumstances. IMAGEN participants underwent the same comprehensive evaluation twice, at age 14 years and at age 19 years thus enabling us to identify factors associated with brain structure at baseline and also with developmental brain changes over the inter-scan interval. We hypothesised that the patterns of covariation identified here would largely follow a "positive-negative" axis of covariation previously shown in studies of young adults (30-32), which have also emphasised that negative influences of social adversity and substance exposure amongst environmental factors. Our aim was to quantify, in the same integrative model, the contribution of biological programmed variables (i.e., age and sex) and variables relating to personal, social and environmental factors.

4.2 Study 3 Methods

4.2.1 Participants

We used data from IMAGEN participants evaluated at age 14 years (baseline) and at age 19 years (developmental change) in eight sites in England, France, Germany and Ireland. At each evaluation, participants had a structural magnetic resonance imaging (MRI) scan and a comprehensive assessment of their individual, social and family characteristics. Following strict quality control procedures, outlined in Figure S1, we selected those participants for whom high-quality imaging data were available at baseline (baseline sample: n=1476) and at both baseline and follow-up assessments (developmental change sample: n=714). Written informed consent was obtained from all participants as well as from their legal guardians. The study was approved by all local ethics committees separately. Table 1 and Supplemental Table S1 summarize the characteristics of participants at baseline and in the developmental change sample.

Table 4.1. Non-imaging characteristics the total analysis sample and the developmental change subsample at their baseline assessment

Variable	Analysis Sample (N=1476)	Developmental Change Subsample (N=714)
Youth Demographic and Anthropometric Features		
Sex (female)	819 (55%)	445 (62%)
Age (years)	14.45 (0.40)	14.45 (0.41)
Height (cm)	167.37 (7.86)	167.32 (7.81)
Weight (kg)	58.23 (10.92)	57.58 (10.29)
Body Mass Index	20.72 (3.24)	20.5 (2.99)
Pubertal Development Scale	13.07 (2.22)	13.2 (2.2)
Youth Perinatal Events		
Birth Weight (grams)	3424 (563)	3419 (553)

Table 4.1. Non-imaging characteristics the total analysis sample and the developmental change subsample at their baseline assessment

Variable	Analysis Sample (N=1476)	Developmental Change Subsample (N=714)
Maternal Smoking During Pregnancy	178 (15%)	76 (12%)
Paternal Smoking During Pregnancy	250 (21%)	108 (18%)
Maternal Alcohol Use During Pregnancy	269 (22%)	142 (23%)
Maternal Medical Illness During Pregnancy	91 (7%)	51 (8%)
Pregnancy and/or Birth Complications	230 (19%)	117 (19%)
Breastfed	1032 (84%)	535 (86%)
Youth Mental Health		
Presence of Psychiatric Diagnosis	192 (13%)	79 (11%)
Youth Cognitive Ability		
General Intelligence g-factor (z-score)	0.02 (0.97)	0.17 (0.88)
ESPAD: Average Grade		
• 1: C-	12 (1%)	2 (0.3%)
• 2: C	28 (2%)	10 (2%)
• 3: C+	40 (3%)	17 (3%)
• 4: B-	48 (4%)	18 (3%)
• 5: B	131 (10%)	59 (9%)
• 6: B+	408 (32%)	178 (29%)
• 7: A-	444 (35%)	244 (39%)
• 8: A	150 (12%)	92 (15%)
ESPAD: Truancy	4.13 (1.56)	3.99 (1.69)
Youth Personality and Temperament		
NEO: Neuroticism	1.88(0.58)	1.91 (0.57)
NEO: Extroversion	2.45(0.43)	2.43 (0.44)
NEO: Openness	2.2(0.47)	2.24 (0.49)
NEO: Agreeableness	2.33(0.4)	2.38 (0.4)
NEO: Conscientiousness	2.3(0.55)	2.36 (0.56)
DAWBA Social Aptitude Scale	24.43(5.79)	24.61 (5.6)
TCI: Novelty Seeking	111.22 (10.42)	110.63 (10.47)
Youth Substance Risk and Use		
SURPS: Anxiety Sensitivity	2.25(0.46)	2.26 (0.46)
SURPS: Hopelessness	1.87(0.41)	1.87 (0.42)
SURPS: Impulsivity	2.43(0.44)	2.39 (0.44)
SURPS: Sensation Seeking	2.77 (0.55)	2.74 (0.54)
ESPAD: Frequency of Lifetime Smoking		
• 0: Never	875 (69%)	459 (74%)
• 1: 1-2 times	178 (14%)	86 (14%)

Table 4.1. Non-imaging characteristics the total analysis sample and the developmental change subsample at their baseline assessment

Variable	Analysis Sample (N=1476)	Developmental Change Subsample (N=714)
• 2: 3-5 times	52 (4%)	19 (3%)
• 3: 6-9 times	40 (3%)	15 (2%)
• 4: 10-19 times	38 (3%)	16 (3%)
• 5: 20-39 times	18 (1%)	10 (2%)
• 6: 40 or more times	60 (5%)	15 (2%)
ESPAD: Smoking in the preceding 30 days		
• 0: Not at all	1127 (89%)	571 (92%)
• 1: less than 1 cigarette per week	56 (4%)	26 (4%)
• 2: less than 1 cigarette per day	28 (2%)	9 (1%)
• 3: 1-5 cigarettes per day	32 (2%)	8 (1%)
• 4: 6-10 cigarettes per day	9 (1%)	3 (0.5%)
• 5: 11-20 cigarettes per day	6 (0.5%)	3 (0.5%)
• 6: more than 20 cigarettes per day	3 (0.2%)	0 (0%)
ESPAD: Frequency of Lifetime Alcohol Use		
• 0: Never	285 (23%)	135 (22%)
• 1: 1-2 times	324 (26%)	161 (26%)
• 2: 3-5 times	239 (19%)	127 (21%)
• 3: 6-9 times	173 (14%)	86 (14%)
• 4: 10-19 times	132 (10%)	68 (11%)
• 5: 20-39 times	64 (5%)	24 (4%)
• 6: 40 or more times	41 (3%)	17 (3%)
ESPAD: Frequency of Alcohol Use in the Preceding 30 Days	638 (51%)	325 (53%)
• 0: Not at al	452 (36%)	218 (35%)
• 1-2 times	104 (8%)	46 (7%)
• 3-5 times	36 (3%)	16 (3%)
• 6-9 times	19 (1%)	10 (2%)
• 10-19 times	6 (0.5%)	2 (0.3%)
• 20-39 times	3 (0.2%)	1 (0.2%)
• 40 or more times		
ESPAD: Frequency of Lifetime Cannabis Use		
• 0: Never	1180 (94%)	592 (96%)
• 1: 1-2 times	41 (3%)	16 (3%)
• 2: 3-5 times	9 (1%)	3 (0.5%)
• 3: 6-9 times	8 (1%)	2 (0.3%)
• 4: 10-19 times		

Table 4.1. Non-imaging characteristics the total analysis sample and the developmental change subsample at their baseline assessment

Variable	Analysis Sample (N=1476)	Developmental Change Subsample (N=714)
• 5: 20-39 times	5 (0.3%)	0 (0%)
• 6: 40 or more times	1 (0.1%)	0 (0%)
	10 (1%)	3 (0.5%)
ESPAD: Frequency of Cannabis Use in the Preceding 30 Days	1211 (96%)	603 (98%)
• 0: 0	30 (2%)	11 (2%)
• 1: 1-2 times	2 (0.2%)	0 (0%)
• 2: 3-5 times	4 (0.3%)	0 (0%)
• 3: 6-9 times	3 (0.2%)	0 (0%)
• 4: 10-19 times	1 (0.1%)	0 (0%)
• 5: 20-39 times	3 (0.2%)	2 (0.3%)
• 6: 40 or more times		
Youth Social and Family Circumstances		
LEQ: Total Number of Negative Life Events since last visit	5.83 (2.96)	5.66 (3.03)
LEQ: Family-related life events since last visit	0.26 (0.23)	0.24 (0.22)
LEQ: Family accidents or illness since last visit	0.53 (0.27)	0.51 (0.27)
LEQ: Events relating to sexuality/intimacy since last visit	0.29 (0.18)	0.28 (0.18)
LEQ: Autonomy: events relating to independence since last visit	0.53 (0.18)	0.53 (0.17)
LEQ: Deviance: events relating to legal or school problems	0.27 (0.23)	0.24 (0.23)
LEQ: Relocation: events relating to change in schools or residence since last visit	0.45 (0.33)	0.45 (0.33)
LEQ: Distress: distressing events since last visit	0.29 (0.19)	0.28 (0.19)
LEQ: Other events since last visit	0.33 (0.27)	0.34 (0.28)
ESPAD: Victim of Bullying	0.19(0.39)	0.2 (0.4)
ESPAD: Perpetrator of Bullying	0.1(0.3)	0.07 (0.26)
DAWBA: Family Stressors: Financial/Housing	0.72(1.08)	0.65 (1.03)
DAWBA: Family Stressors: Work Pressure	1.07(1.08)	1.11 (1.09)
DAWBA: Family Stressors: Illness	0.52(0.9)	0.51 (0.9)
DAWBA: Family Stressors: Relationships/Addiction	0.42(0.74)	0.39 (0.73)
DAWBA: Child Experience: Affirmation	10.82(1.47)	10.9 (1.35)
DAWBA: Child Experience: Discipline	3.43(1.58)	3.35 (1.58)
DAWBA: Child Experience: Rules	4.64(1.24)	4.64 (1.27)
DAWBA: Living With Both Parents	1267 (86%)	620 (87%)

Table 4.1. Non-imaging characteristics the total analysis sample and the developmental change subsample at their baseline assessment

Variable	Analysis Sample (N=1476)	Developmental Change Subsample (N=714)
FIGS: Positive Family History of Psychiatric Disorders	274 (19%)	129 (18%)
Parental Characteristics		
ESPAD: Maternal Education Level		
• GCSEs or CSEs or below	235 (17%)	90 (13%)
• NVQ or GNVQ	273 (19%)	112 (16%)
• A levels or a BTEC national diploma	204 (15%)	111 (16%)
• Advanced diploma	203 (14%)	100 (15%)
• Bachelor degree	321 (23%)	175 (26%)
• Professional Qualification (Master's degree and above)	162 (11%)	91 (13%)
ESPAD: Paternal Education Level		
• GCSEs or CSEs or below	300 (21%)	113 (17%)
• GNVQ or NVQ	209 (15%)	109 (16%)
• A levels or a BTEC national diploma	175 (12%)	86 (13%)
• Advanced diploma	164 (12%)	78 (12%)
• Bachelor degree	313 (22%)	168 (25%)
• Professional Qualification (Master's degree and above)	237 (17%)	125 (18%)

Continuous variables are shown as mean (standard deviation); categorical variables are shown as number (percentage;%); ESPAD= European School Survey Project on Alcohol and Other Drugs; DAWBA=Development and Well-being Assessment; FIGS: Family Interview for Genetic Studies; LEQ=Life Events Questionnaire; NEO= NEO-Five Factor Personality Inventory; SURPS=Substance Use Risk Profile Scale; TCI=Temperament and Character Inventory; WISC-IV=Wechsler Intelligence Scale for Children-IV; GCSE=General Certificate of Secondary Education; CSE= Certificate of Secondary Education; GNVC= General National Vocational Qualification; NVQ= National Vocational Qualification; BTEC=Business and Technology Education Council; A levels=Advanced Level Qualification; Details of each variable are shown in Supplemental Table S2.

4.2.2 Non-imaging Variables

We considered variables corresponding to youths' demographic characteristics (age and sex), anthropomorphic features (height, weight, body mass index and pubertal stage), perinatal events (parental smoking/substance use, maternal medical conditions, birth complications, breastfeeding), mental health (presence or absence of psychiatric diagnoses), cognitive ability (general intelligence and scholastic performance), personality and temperament, substance use and risk, social and family circumstances (life events, bullying, family function, socioeconomic status, housing) and parental education level. Because our study focuses on general neurodevelopment, we didn't include measures of individual psychopathologies (interested reader is referred to the paper by Ing et al. on that topic[167], a full list of IMAGEN publications is provided in the supplementary material). Definitions of the variables and description of the assessment instruments are presented in Supplemental Table S2. Missing values for non-imaging features were imputed using random forest in R using available values from other non-imaging features (package missForest version 1.4) although the percentage of missing values was generally low (Supplemental Table S3).

4.2.3 Neuroimaging Acquisition and Processing

High-resolution T_1-weighted images were obtained at eight European sites (Berlin, Dresden, Dublin, Hamburg, London, Mannheim, Nottingham and Paris) with 3T MRI systems by different manufacturers (Siemens: 4 sites, Philips: 2 sites, General Electric: 1 site, and Bruker: 1 site). The MR protocols, cross-site standardization and quality control procedures of the IMAGEN study are described in the supplemental material and in Schumann et al (2010)[168]. In addition to the standard IMAGEN procedures we also applied a validated automatic quality control algorithm (Qoala-T;

(https://github.com/Qoala-T/QC) [169] to preprocessed MRI scans to exclude low quality images at each assessment wave (Supplemental Figure S1). Subsequently, we used an automatic robust longitudinal processing pipeline [170] to extract reliable estimates of cortical thickness and surface area and subcortical volumes (Supplemental Table S4) using Freesurfer version 6.0 (https://surfer.nmr.mgh.harvard.edu/). The final baseline (n=1476) and developmental change (n=714) samples were defined following outlier exclusion undertaken in each sample separately using the Mahalanobis distance with a quantile cut-off of 0.999 implemented in chemometrics package, version 1.4.2, in R. Prior to statistical analysis, the imaging variables were adjusted for site/scanner effects using ComBat in R (https://github.com/Jfortin1/ComBatHarmonization) [71]. Initially used for batch adjustment of genetic data, ComBat uses Empirical Bayes to adjust for between-site variability while preserving biological variability.

4.2.4 Statistical Analysis

4.2.4.1 Descriptive Statistics: For all variables, differences in baseline and follow-up values were examined using paired t-tests or McNemar's tests for continuous and categorical variables respectively.

4.2.4.2 Datasets: The neuroimaging and non-imaging datasets and their constituent variables were described above and in the supplementary tables S2 and S4. Cortical thickness, cortical surface area, and subcortical volumes were examined separately because these phenotypes are genetically independent and follow different developmental trajectories[35,171,172]. Analyses of the baseline sample (n=1476) were included

global neuroimaging measures (e.g., mean cortical thickness, total surface area, and total

intracranial volume). Values of brain regional measures for each imaging phenotype

(cortical thickness, area and subcortical volume) were thus not adjusted by their

respective global measures. In the developmental change subsample (n=714) we were

interested in modeling the effect on the variables that changed between the baseline and

follow-up assessments. In each IMAGEN participant, developmental change in any

variable was calculated as: (follow-up value – baseline value) which was then

residualized by the baseline value. Parental education and perinatal events were not

included in the developmental change analyses as their values did not change between

baseline and follow-up. Pubertal development and general intelligence (g-factor) were

not included in the main developmental change analyses these were not assessed at

follow up. We also performed additional sCCA on the developmental change data with

these variables included. Sex was retained in the main model as it exerts a continuous

influence on brain structural development during adolescence.

4.2.4.3 Identification of multivariate associations between imaging and non-imaging

datasets: We used sparse canonical correlations analyses[166], which is a version of the

general canonical correlation analysis (CCA), to identify linked dimensions between

imaging and the non-imaging datasets (additional details in the supplementary material).

Canonical correlation analysis (CCA) is a method for finding relationships between two multivariate sets of variables, all measured in the same individuals[166]. CCA seeks to find

linear combinations of variables from each dataset that express maximal correlation

between the two datasets (referred to as pairs of canonical variates or modes). Traditional

CCA models are prone to overfitting and are not fully equipped to deal with variables

that are correlated. Regularization is commonly employed to penalize the complexity of

a learning model and control overfitting. Sparse CCA (sCCA) implements regularization

by using a sparsity parameter which penalizes some variables by setting their

contribution to the overall model to zero. In addition to the pairs of variates (i.e., one

variate from each dataset), sCCA generates information for variables with non-zero

contributions. These are expressed as weights (i.e., magnitude of the contribution of the

variable to the variate from the same dataset) and as canonical cross-loadings (i.e.,

coefficient of the correlation of the variable with the variate of the opposite dataset).

In this study, sCCA models were implemented in R version 6.8.0 using the

sgcca.wrapper function from the mixOmics package (version 6.14.0). Non-imaging and

neuroimaging variables were standardized to a mean of 0 and a standard deviation of 1

before being entered into the sCCA models[166,173]. We then followed standard procedures

to identify the optimal sparsity parameters for each sCCA model. For each analysis, we

computed the sparse parameters by running the sCCA with a range of candidate values

(from $1/\sqrt{p}$ to 1, at 10 increments, where p is the number of features in that view of the

data) for each imaging and non-imaging dataset, and then fitted the resulting models. We selected the optimal sparse criteria combination based on the parameters that corresponded to the values of the model that maximized the sCCA correlation value. We then computed the optimal sCCA model and determined its significance based on exact P-values calculated from 1000 random permutations. The p-value was defined as the number of permutations that resulted in an equal or higher correlation than the original data divided by the total number of permutations (further details in Supplemental material). Because we implemented multiple sCCA models throughout the manuscript, significance of each mode was further adjusted using false discovery correction (FDR). In addition, statistically significant modes were tested for reliability and reproducibility (described below) and only models that survived these analyses are reported. For significant sCCA mode, we report weights and loadings of the contributing variables if these are at least of small effect (>|0.1|) according to current standards [174].

4.2.4.4 Reliability, Reproducibility and Supplemental Analyses: We undertook the following analyses to determine the robustness of our results: (i) we tested the association between image quality and canonical correlation coefficients. A quality score for each individual scan was calculated using the Qoala algorithm. We then computed the spearman's correlation coefficient between the mean data quality score and the sCCA - coefficients derived from 500 randomly resampled subsets of the original sample; (ii) we assessed the stability of the findings of each sCCA in relation to sample size and composition. To do so we repeated each sCCA in 100 randomly generated subsets each containing 10 to 150% of the original data in 10% increments (1500 subsamples in total); (iii) following our prior work [161], we calculated redundancy reliability (RR) scores for each sCCA ; to achieve this we repeated each sCCA in 500 randomly generated subsets and quantified the reliability of canonical cross loadings (details in supplemental material); (iv) we randomly sampled 50% of the data 500 times (training set), calculated sCCA on each training set and then used the weights from the sCCA on the training set on the remainder 50% of the data (test set) to calculate the canonical correlations in the test set. We reported only those modes that met the following robustness criteria: (i) statistically significant at an FDR-corrected P-value<0.001; (ii) had a median RR-score>0.80, and (iii) average canonical correlation on the resampled test sets was at least 80% of that of the training sets. We performed additional sCCAs to evaluate the effect of removing sex and age on the results.

4.2.4.5 Code Availability: Analysis code is available at

https://github.com/AmirhosseinModabbernia/IMAGEN

4.3 Study 3 Results

The non-imaging characteristics of the baseline sample and developmental change subsample are shown in Table 1 and Supplemental Table S1. The corresponding descriptive statistics for cortical thickness and area and subcortical volumes are presented in Supplemental Table S5. At a nominal statistical level, the follow-up subsample included more women (P<0.001) and more offspring of parents with higher levels of parental education (P<0.05) than the baseline sample (Table 1). Over the 5-year mean inter-scan interval, the mean (standard deviation, SD) of the global cortical thickness decreased by 0.12(0.06) mm on the right and 0.13(0.06) mm on the left. Total cortical surface area showed an average decrease of 3891(2274) mm² during the same period.

4.3.1 Linked imaging and non-imaging dimensions

4.3.1.1 Cortical Thickness: 4.3.1.1.1 Baseline: The sCCA testing the association between cortical thickness measures and non-imaging variables was significant (r =0.30, P_{FDR}<0.001, mean (SD) permuted r=0.12(0.01)) (Figure 1A) and accounted for 9% of the covariance (Supplemental Figures S2). The canonical weights and cross-loadings for the imaging and non-imaging variables are shown in Supplemental Tables S6 to S9. Sex and age had the highest positive canonical cross-loadings on the imaging variate while the frequency of negative family life events had the highest negative canonical cross-loading (Figure 1B; supplemental Table S7). Canonical cross-loadings of ϱ>0.10 were noted for nearly all cortical regions and were highest for the mean total cortical thickness and for the rostral middle frontal cortex (Figure 1C; Supplemental Table S9). 4.3.1.1.2 Developmental change: The sCCA testing the association between developmental changes in cortical thickness measures and inter-scan changes in non-imaging variables was significant (r =0.34, P_{FDR}<0.001, mean (SD) permuted r=0.16(0.02)) (Figure 1D) and accounted for 12% of the covariance (Supplemental Figures S3). The canonical weights and cross-loadings for the imaging and non-imaging variables are shown in Supplemental Tables S10 to S13. Inter-scan changes in age, height, and frequency of alcohol and cannabis use had the highest negative canonical cross-loadings (Figure 1E; Supplemental Table S11). Developmental changes in cortical thickness with canonical cross-loadings of $\varrho > 0.1$ were noted in most cortical regions; the highest loadings were found in the superior frontal, the pars opercularis, supramarginal, bank of the superior temporal sulcus, and posterior cingulate cortices (Figure 1F; Supplemental Table S13).

4.3.1.2 Cortical Surface Area: <u>4.3.1.2.1 Baseline</u>: The sCCA testing for the association between cortical surface area measures and non-imaging variables was significant (r =0.62, $P_{FDR}<0.001$, mean (SD) permuted r=0.12(0.01)) (Figure 2A) and accounted for 38%

of the covariance (Supplemental Figures S4). The canonical weights and cross-loadings

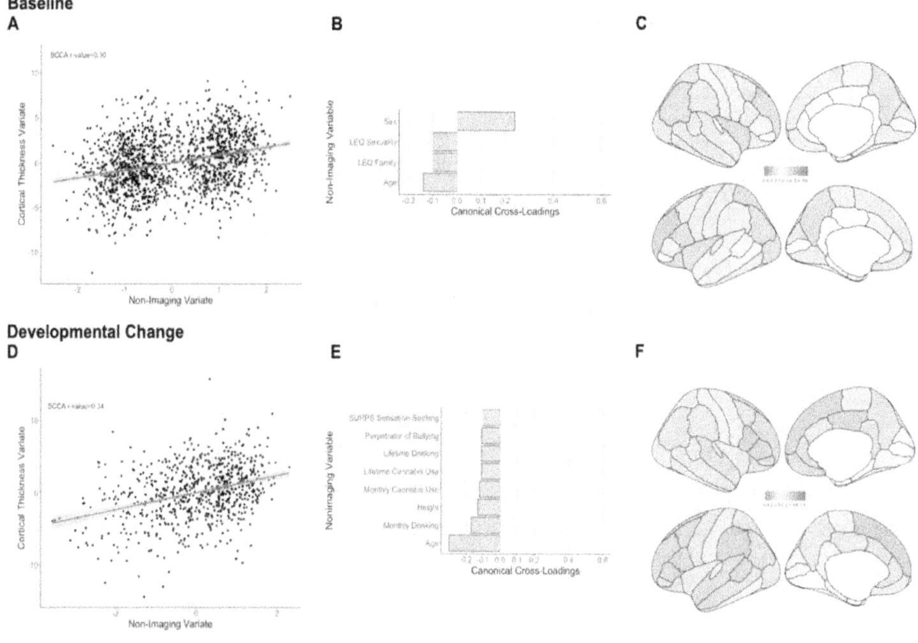

Figure 4.1: Sparse canonical correlation analysis (sCCA) for baseline and developmental change in cortical thickness.
Upper panel: Baseline: **a** First canonical correlation coefficient. **b** Canonical cross-loadings for non-imaging variables. **c** Canonical cross-loadings for imaging variables. Lower panel: Developmental change: **d** First canonical correlation coefficient. **e** Canonical cross-loadings for non-imaging variables. **f** Canonical cross-loadings for imaging variables. LEQ Life Event Questionnaire, SURPS Substance Use Risk Profile Scale.

for the imaging and non-imaging variables are shown in supplemental Tables S14 to S17.

The highest positive canonical cross-loadings were observed for sex, anthropometric measures (height, weight and birthweight), youth cognitive ability and parental education. The highest negative canonical cross-loadings were observed for youth neuroticism and anxiety sensitivity and parental perinatal smoking (Figure 2B; supplemental Table S15). Canonical cross-loadings with the non-imaging variate with ϱ

values ranging from 0.20 to 0.60 were noted for all cortical regions with the top five seen for the total surface area, and the surface area of the left superior temporal cortex the left rostral middle frontal cortex, the right fusiform and the right insula (ϱ=0.50-0.60) (Figure 2C; supplemental Table S17). 4.3.1.2.2 Developmental Change: The sCCA testing the association between developmental changes in cortical surface area and inter-scan changes in non-imaging variables was significant (r =0.59, P_{FDR}<0.001, mean (SD) permuted r=0.20(0.02)) (Figure 2D) and accounted for 35% of the covariance (Supplemental Figures S5). The canonical weights and cross-loadings for the imaging inter-scan changes in age and in anthropometric features (height and weight), cannabis use, and sensation seeking/deviance had the highest positive canonical cross-loadings with the imaging variate whereas anxiety sensitivity, distressing and negative life events had the highest negative canonical cross-loadings (Figure 2E; supplemental Table S19). Developmental changes in the surface area showed mostly positive and non- imaging variables are shown in supplemental Tables S18 to S21. Male sex, and small to moderate canonical cross-loadings (ϱ<0.35) throughout the cortex; notable negative canonical cross-loadings were noted within the bank of the superior temporal gyrus bilaterally (Figure 2F; Supplemental Table S21).

4.3.1.3 Subcortical Volumes: <u>4.3.1.3.1 Baseline</u>: The sCCA testing for the association between subcortical volumes and non-imaging variables was significant (r =0.65, P$_{FDR}$<0.001, mean (SD) permuted r=0.12(0.01)) (Figure 3A) and accounted for 42% of the

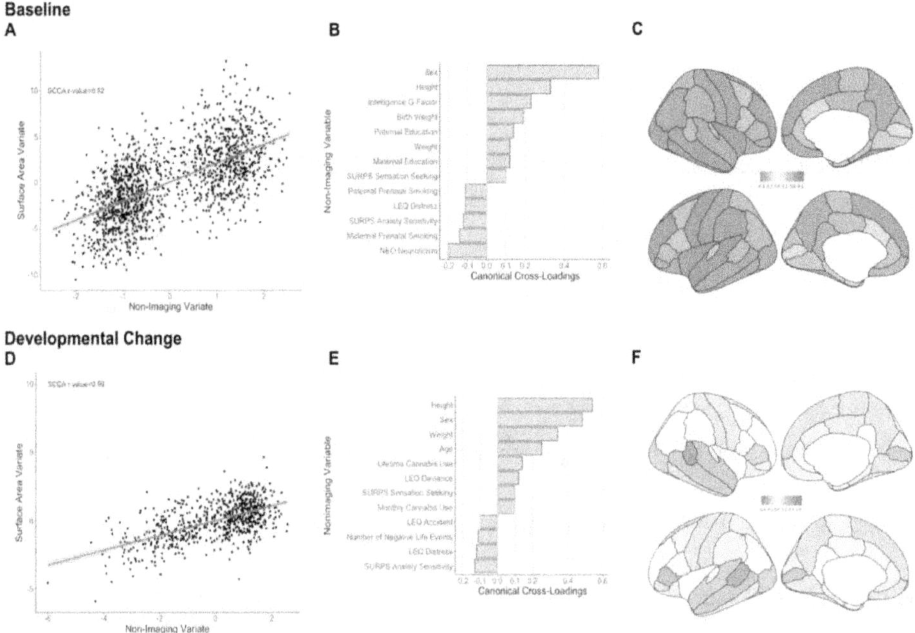

Figure 4.2: Sparse canonical correlation analysis (sCCA) for baseline and developmental change in cortical surface area.
Upper panel: Baseline: **a** First canonical correlation coefficient. **b** Canonical cross-loadings for non-imaging variables. **c** Canonical cross-loadings for imaging variables. Lower panel: Developmental change: **d** First canonical correlation coefficient. **e** Canonical cross-loadings for non-imaging variables. **f** Canonical cross-loadings for imaging variables. LEQ Life Event Questionnaire, SURPS Substance Use Risk Profile Scale, NEO NEO-Five Factor Personality Inventory.

covariance (Supplemental Figures S6). The canonical weights and cross-loadings for the imaging and non-imaging variables are shown in supplemental Tables S22 to S25. Sex, youth's general cognitive ability and anthropometric measures (height, birth weight, and weight) showed the highest positive canonical cross-loadings while maternal prenatal smoking and youth personality traits relating to anxiety and neuroticism showed the highest negative canonical cross-loading (Figure 3B; Supplemental Table S23). Canonical cross-loadings with the non-imaging variate with ϱ values ranging from 0.14 to 0.61 were noted for all subcortical regions with the top five being the total intracranial volume, the cerebellum and the thalamus (Figure 3C; supplemental Table S25). <u>4.3.1.3.2 Developmental Change</u>: The sCCA testing the association between developmental changes in regional subcortical volumes was significant (r =0.54, P_{FDR}<0.001, mean (SD) permuted r=0.18(0.02)) (Figure 3D) and accounted for 29% of the related to sexuality and youth personality traits relating to anxiety and conscientiousness showed the highest negative canonical cross-loadings (Figure 3E; Supplemental Table S27). Developmental changes in regional subcortical volumes with showed positive canonical cross-loadings with ϱ values ranging from 0.10 to 0.40, with lateral ventricles having the smallest canonical cross-loadings (ϱ range 0.10-0.12) (Figure 3F; Supplemental Table S29).

4.3.2 Reliability Analysis

Only the first mode for each sCCA analysis passed the criteria for reporting (Supplemental Figures S2 to S7). Resampling analyses showed that the canonical correlations were largely stable for samples larger than 50% of the originals. The results of the stability and reliability analyses are summarized in Supplemental Figures S8 and S9 and Supplemental Table S30. To quantify the associations beyond the effect of age and sex we also reran the sCCA after regressing out age and sex from both imaging and non-imaging variables. We found that in most cases (except for cortical thickness at baseline), first canonical mode remained significant (Supplemental Table S31). Further sCCA analysis showed that among variables that were only measured at baseline, maternal education, pubertal stage, and history of being breastfed had significant association with

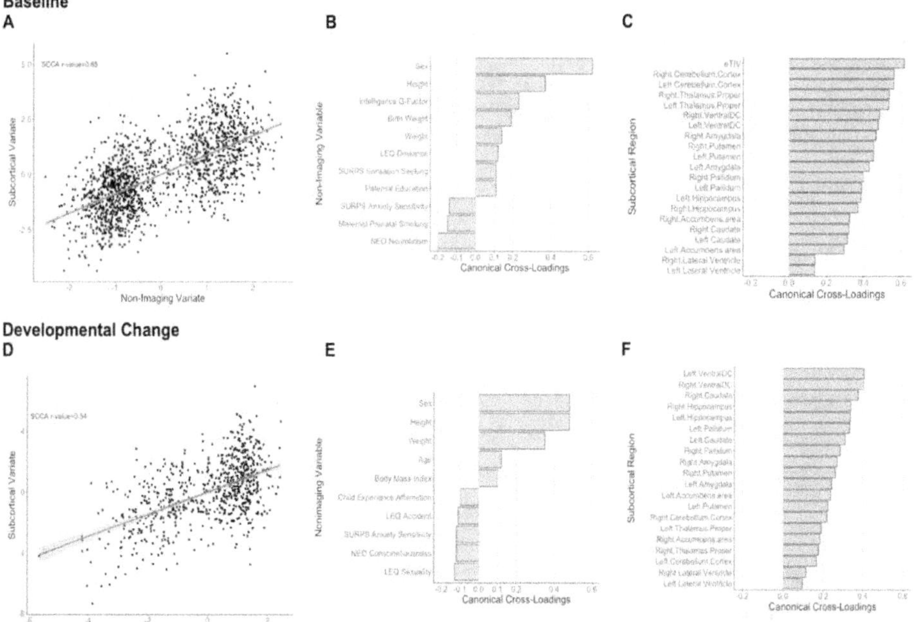

Figure 4.3: Sparse canonical correlation analysis (sCCA) for baseline and developmental change in subcortical volumes.

Upper panel: Baseline: a First canonical correlation coefficient. b Canonical cross-loadings for non-imaging variables. c Canonical cross-loadings for imaging variables. Lower panel: Developmental change: d First canonical correlation coefficient. e Canonical cross-loadings for non-imaging variables. f Canonical cross-loadings for imaging variables. LEQ Life Event Questionnaire, SURPS Substance Use Risk Profile Scale, NEO NEO-Five Factor Personality Inventory.

the imaging variate (Supplemental Table S32).

4.4 Study 3 Discussion

We leveraged the rich dataset and a longitudinal design of the IMAGEN study to identify patterns of covariation between adolescent brain structure and youth personal attributes, lifestyle and psychosocial environment. Using integrated multivariate analyses, we demonstrate that adolescent brain structural development was most strongly associated with sex, age and anthropometric features. Contributions from environmental sources were quantitatively smaller and highlighted the influence of parental smoking and education, unpleasant life events and youths' cognitive ability, use of alcohol and cannabis and personality traits related to negative affect.

We found that measures of cortical thickness, surface area and subcortical volumes show mostly unitary patterns of covariation that reflect the corresponding global measures. Regional and global brain structural measures, both at baseline and at follow-up, showed the highest covariation with sex, age and anthropometric measures. These associations have been consistently noted in prior research [148,161,175]. However, the integrated analyses implemented here enable the study of these factors in the wider context of other potential influences relating to environmental exposures. Thus, a novel finding of the current study is that biologically programmed processes relating to sexual dimorphism and the time-dependent evolution of development remain the most significant drivers of adolescent brain development even when accounting for other influences.

Beyond sex and age, our findings support previous reports in young adults, which have found that the pattern of covariation of brain-derived phenotypes largely recapitulates conventional notions of "positive" and "negative" influences (30, 31). We showed that global surface area and intracranial volume, but not cortical thickness show substantial correlation the overall intelligence (g-factor), thus affirming the association between cognitive abilities and brain organization [176,177]. In line with previous observations, the strength of this association was moderate [178] and more notable at baseline. Schmitt and colleagues (2019) [179] have also reported that beyond the age of 10-11 years, the association between cortical thickness and intelligence is weak. As suggested by others, the relationship between brain structure and cognitive ability might be ever-changing and is likely to be influenced both by baseline brain structure and its dynamic changes over time [180].

A key finding of the current study with important public health implications concerns the "lingering" influence of parental smoking and birth weight for brain structure in adolescence. Cigarette smoking in pregnant women has been associated with premature birth, low birth weight, stillbirth, asthma, learning and behavioral disability, and a predisposition to disease [181]. The mechanisms underlying the relation between perinatal exposure to smoking and brain structure are beyond the resolution of the available data in this study, but we note that maternal smoking has been associated with epigenetic modulation of birthweight [182]. There may be further mechanistic links as smoking has emerged as one of the most powerful epigenetic modulators amongst environmental exposures [183].

Alcohol and cannabis use were associated with accelerated cortical thinning and mild increase in cortical surface area and subcortical volumes. Our findings are generally in line with previous studies [160,161] showing that even the mild substance use commonly encountered in general population is associated with measurable structural changes in the brain although the literature on the specific regions impacted is less consistent [184,185]. Frontoparietal and cingulate cortices had the largest decrease in cortical thickness in relation to substance use and sensation seeking behavior, possibly delineating the critical role of maturational changes in these regions in development of inhibitory control during adolescence [186].

Personality traits associated with anxiety and neuroticism were also associated with smaller surface area in adolescents. Similar results were obtained in young adults participating in the Human Connectome Project; in that study neuroticism was negatively associated with cortical surface area in the left precentral, left superior parietal, left occipital and right superior temporal regions [158]. Some studies have suggested that the association between neuroticism and brain structure is sex-dependent [187]. Our results suggest that this may not be the case in this age-group when multiple other factors are simultaneously modeled. Intriguingly conscientiousness had a negative cross-loading to the variate of subcortical volumes. Conscientiousness has shown positive associations with processing speed[188-191] but negative associations with fluid intelligence[192,193], the latter being associated with larger subcortical volumes[194]. Although speculative, the negative cross-loading of conscientiousness with developmental change in subcortical volume may be aligned with proposal that high level of persistence and dutifulness may compensate for lower general abilities[192,193].

The main strengths of this study include the large sample size, longitudinal design, and rich phenotyping of the IMAGEN cohort. We adopted a robust quality control procedure, where we used a longitudinal image analysis pipeline together with a two-level quality control process. Further, the analytic methods addressed several major issues in population neuroscience including analysis of high dimensional data, stability, and reliability. Study limitations include the exclusive focus on atlas-based measures of brain structure, which provides a common framework for image analysis, but arguably limits the granularity of the data analysis. Structural measures are more reliable than other brain phenotypes but the lack of other brain phenotypes in the current study limits the generalizability of the findings to brain function or connectivity.

In summary, using multivariate statistical techniques, we found multiple reliable correlates of adolescent brain structure. Our study highlights the critical role for programmed biological processes such as indicated by sex, age, measures of physical growth, and intellectual functioning in brain development. Nevertheless, our findings also provide evidence for numerically smaller but statistically robust associations between brain structural phenotypes and modifiable social and environmental influences such as substance use, parental education, and life and perinatal events.

4.5 Study 3 Supplemental Material

Due to very large volume of the supplemental files, important tables and figures are presented below and the rest are available only online. The full supplemental material for this study can be accessed online through the following links: https://static-content.springer.com/esm/art%3A10.1038%2Fs41380-020-0757-x/MediaObjects/41380_2020_757_MOESM1_ESM.docx

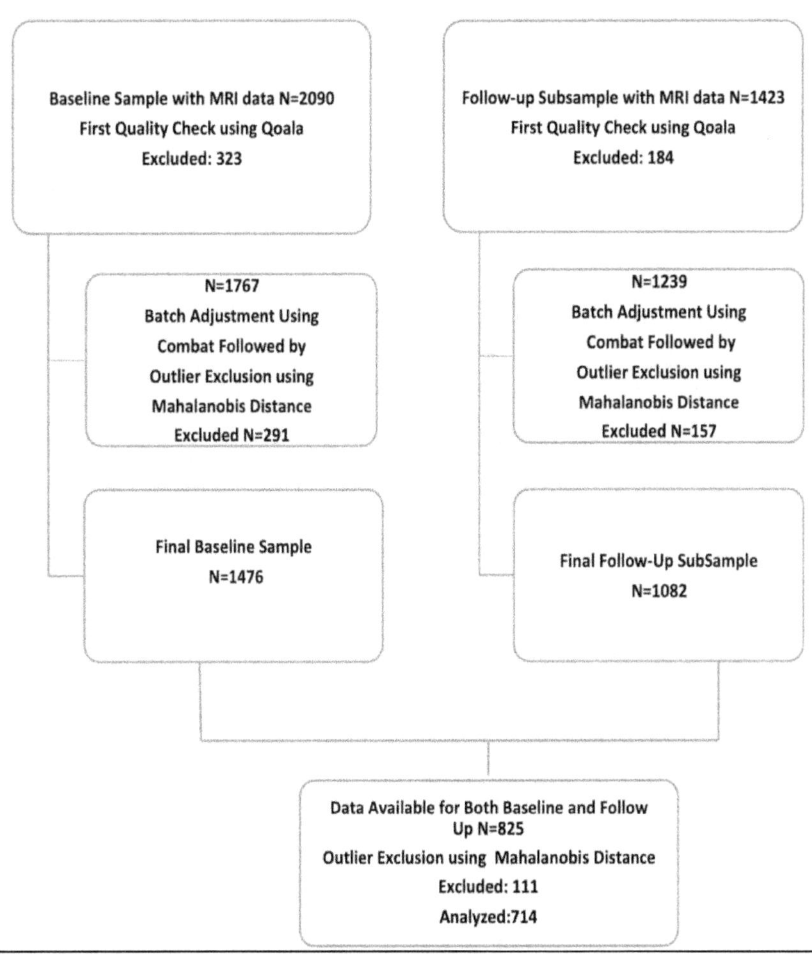

Figure S1. Flowchart for Participant selection from the IMAGEN cohort

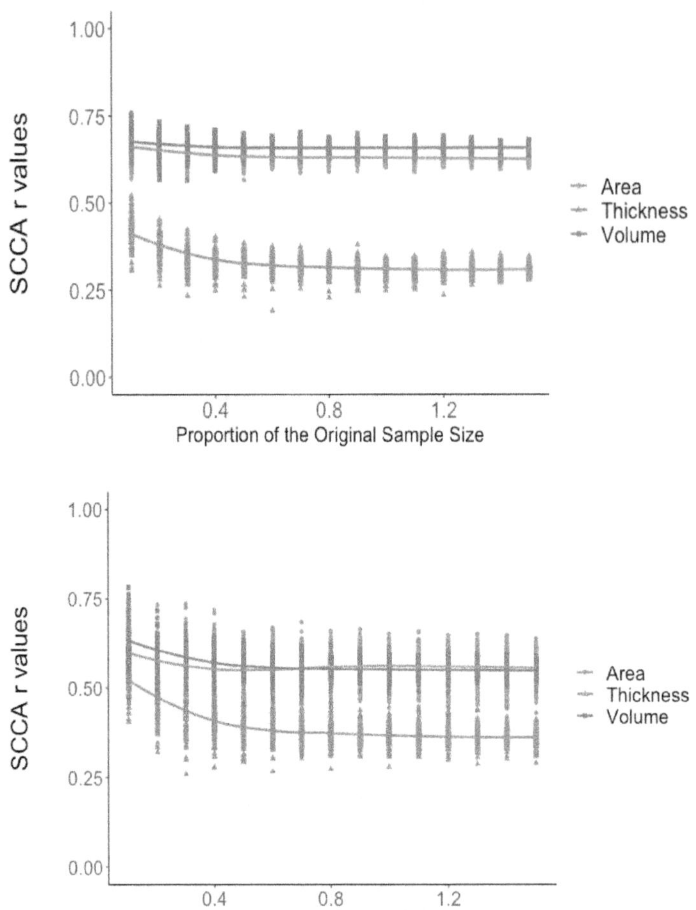

Figure S8. Reliability of the results as a function of sample size
A. Baseline B. Developmental Change

Table S1. Changes in the developmental change subsample (n=714) between their baseline and follow-up assessments

Variable	Baseline Assessment	Follow-up Assessment
Youth Demographic and Anthropometric Features		
Sex (female)	445 (62%)	-
Age (years)*	14.45 (0.41)	19.07 (0.75)
Height (cm)*	167.32 (7.81)	172.31 (9.14)
Weight (kg)*	57.58 (10.29)	66.61 (12.45)
Body Mass Index*	20.5 (2.99)	22.37 (3.47)

Physical Development Scale	13.2 (2.2)	-
Youth Perinatal Events		
Birth Weight (grams)	3419 (553)	-
Maternal Smoking During Pregnancy	76 (12%)	-
Paternal Smoking During Pregnancy	108 (18%)	-
Maternal Alcohol Use During Pregnancy	142 (23%)	-
Maternal Medical Illness During Pregnancy	51 (8%)	-
Pregnancy and/or Birth Complications	117 (19%)	-
Breastfed	535 (86%)	-
Youth Mental Health		
Psychiatric Diagnosis*	79 (11%)	99 (14%)
Youth Cognitive Ability		
General Intelligence (g-factor), Z-Score	0.17 (0.88)	-
ESPAD: Average Grade		
• 1: C-	2 (0.3%)	9 (1%)
• 2: C	10 (2%)	7 (1%)
• 3: C+	17 (3%)	21 (3%)
• 4: B-	18 (3%)	28 (4%)
• 5: B	59 (9%)	53 (9%)
• 6: B+	178 (29%)	192 (31%)
• 7: A-	244 (39%)	210 (34%)
• 8: A	92 (15%)	99 (16%)
ESPAD: Truancy*	3.99 (1.69)	4.19 (1.86)
Youth Personality and Temperament		
NEO: Neuroticism*[195]	1.91 (0.57)	1.71 (0.66)
NEO: Extroversion	2.43 (0.44)	2.41 (0.45)
NEO: Openness*	2.24 (0.49)	2.36 (0.51)
NEO: Agreeableness*	2.38 (0.4)	2.56 (0.42)
NEO: Conscientiousness*	2.36 (0.56)	2.51 (0.61)
DAWBA Social Aptitude Scale*	24.61 (5.6)	25.61 (6.25)
TCI: Novelty Seeking*	110.63 (10.47)	107.12 (10.76)
Youth Substance Risk and Use		
SURPS: Anxiety Sensitivity*	2.26 (0.46)	2.35 (0.46)
SURPS: Hopelessness	1.87 (0.42)	1.86 (0.47)
SURPS: Impulsivity*	2.39 (0.44)	2.19 (0.41)
SURPS: Sensation Seeking	2.74 (0.54)	2.78 (0.54)
ESPAD Frequency of ESPAD Frequency of Lifetime Smoking*		
• 0: 0	459 (74%)	196 (32%)
• 1: 1-2 times	86 (14%)	77 (12%)
• 2: 3-5 times	19 (3%)	61 (10%)
• 3: 6-9 times	15 (2%)	30 (5%)
• 4: 10-19 times	16 (3%)	45 (8%)
• 5: 20-39 times	10 (2%)	28 (4%)
• 6: 40 or more times	15 (2%)	182 (29%)

ESPAD: Smoking the preceding 30 days*

• 0: Not at all	571 (92%)	384 (62%)
• 1: less than 1 cigarette per week	26 (4%)	65 (10%)
• 2: less than 1 cigarette per day	9 (1%)	42 (7%)
• 3: 1-5 cigarettes per day	8 (1%)	49 (8%)
• 4: 6-10 cigarettes per day	3 (0.5%)	45 (7%)
• 5: 11-20 cigarettes per day	3 (0.5%)	30 (5%)
• 6: more than 20 cigarettes per day	0 (0%)	4 (1%)

ESPAD: Lifetime Alcohol Use*

• 0: 0	135 (22%)	15 (2%)
• 1: 1-2 times	161 (26%)	15 (2%)
• 2: 3-5 times	127 (21%)	24 (4%)
• 3: 6-9 times	86 (14%)	37 (6%)
• 4: 10-19 times	68 (11%)	67 (11%)
• 5: 20-39 times	24 (4%)	106 (17%)
• 6: 40 or more times	17 (3%)	355 (57%)

ESPAD: Alcohol Use in the preceding 30 days*

• 0: 0	325 (53%)	54 (9%)
• 1-2 times	218 (35%)	194 (31%)
• 3-5 times	46 (7%)	153 (25%)
• 6-9 times	16 (3%)	113 (18%)
• 10-19 times	10 (2%)	72 (12%)
• 20-39 times	2 (0.3%)	20 (3%)
• 40 or more times	1 (0.2%)	13 (2%)

ESPAD Frequency of Lifetime Cannabis use *

• 0: 0	592 (96%)	320 (52%)
• 1: 1-2 times	16 (3%)	65 (11%)
• 2: 3-5 times	3 (0.5%)	48 (8%)
• 3: 6-9 times	2 (0.3%)	40 (6%)
• 4: 10-19 times	0 (0%)	35 (6%)
• 5: 20-39 times	0 (0%)	32 (5%)
• 6: 40 or more times	3 (0.5%)	78 (13%)

ESPAD: Cannabis Use in the preceding 30 days*

• 0: 0	603 (98%)	347 (56%)
• 1: 1-2 times	11 (2%)	116 (19%)
• 2: 3-5 times	0 (0%)	51 (8%)
• 3: 6-9 times	0 (0%)	33 (5%)
• 4: 10-19 times	0 (0%)	33 (5%)
• 5: 20-39 times	0 (0%)	22 (4%)
• 6: 40 or more times	2 (0.3%)	16 (3%)

Youth Social and Family Circumstances		
LEQ: Number of Negative Life Events*	5.66 (3.03)	3.19 (2.29)
LEQ: Family*	0.24 (0.22)	0.13 (0.17)
LEQ: Accident*	0.51 (0.27)	0.35 (0.26)
LEQ: Sexuality*	0.28 (0.18)	0.35 (0.21)
LEQ: Autonomy*	0.53 (0.17)	0.6 (0.19)
LEQ: Deviance*	0.24 (0.23)	0.09 (0.19)
LEQ: Relocation*	0.45 (0.33)	0.11 (0.19)

LEQ: Distress*	0.28 (0.19)	0.21 (0.18)
LEQ: Other*	0.34 (0.28)	0.29 (0.24)
ESPAD: Victim of Bullying*	0.2 (0.4)	0.04 (0.21)
ESPAD: Perpetrator of Bullying*	0.07 (0.26)	0.01 (0.13)
DAWBA: Family Stressors: Financial/Housing	0.65 (1.03)	0.59 (1.02)
DAWBA: Family Stressors: Work/Pressure*	1.11 (1.09)	1.01 (1.08)
DAWBA: Family Stressors: Illness	0.51 (0.9)	0.55 (0.94)
DAWBA: Family Stressors Relationships/Addiction	0.39 (0.73)	0.39 (0.7)
DAWBA: Child Experience: Affirmation	10.9 (1.35)	10.93 (1.36)
DAWBA: Child Experience: Discipline*	3.35 (1.58)	2.96 (1.5)
DAWBA: Child Experience: Rules	4.64 (1.27)	4.67 (1.26)
DAWBA: Living With Both Parents*	620 (87%)	554 (88%)
FIGS: Positive Family History of Psychiatric Disorders	129 (18%)	-
Parental Characteristics		
ESPAD: Maternal Education Level		
• GCSEs or CSEs or below	90 (13%)	-
• NVQ or GNVQ	112 (16%)	-
• A levels or a BTEC national diploma	111 (16%)	-
• Advanced diploma	100 (15%)	-
• Bachelor degree	175 (26%)	-
• Professional Qualifications (Master's degree and above)	91 (13%)	-
ESPAD: Paternal Education Level		
• GCSEs or CSEs or below	113 (17%)	-
• NVQ or GNVQ	109 (16%)	-
• A levels or a BTEC national diploma	86 (13%)	-
• Advanced diploma	78 (12%)	-
• Bachelor degree	168 (25%)	-
• Professional Qualifications (Master's degree and above)	125 (18%)	-

* Denotes differences between baseline and follow-up at P<0.05 uncorrected; Continuous variables are shown as mean (standard deviation); categorical variables are shown as number (percentage;%); follow-up LEQ values are mean number of life events happening after the last visit. ESPAD= European School Survey Project on Alcohol and Other Drugs; DAWBA=Development and Well-being Assessment; FIGS: Family Interview for Genetic Studies; LEQ=Life Events Questionnaire; NEO= NEO-Five Factor Personality Inventory; SURPS=Substance Use Risk Profile Scale; TCI=Temperament and Character Inventory; WISC-IV=Wechsler Intelligence Scale for Children-IV; GCSE=General Certificate of Secondary Education; CSE= Certificate of Secondary Education; GNVC= General National Vocational Qualification; NVQ= National Vocational Qualification; BTEC= Business and Technology Education Council; A levels=Advance Level Qualification. Details on each variable in Supplemental Table S2 and S3.

115

Table S30. Mean and standard deviations of supplemental Correlation coefficients for the first five modes in 500 test/train sets

	Baseline					
Modes	Thickness		Surface Area		Volume	
	Train	Test	Train	Test	Train	Test
1	0.28(0.01)	0.26(0.03)	0.62(0.01)	0.62(0.02)	0.65(0.01)	0.65(0.02)
2	0.19(0.03)	0.11(0.05)	0.12(0.04)	0.02(0.06)	0.2(0.06)	0.17(0.08)
3	0.15(0.03)	0.07(0.05)	0.14(0.04)	0.05(0.07)	0.1(0.07)	0.05(0.09)
4	0.15(0.03)	0.06(0.05)	0.14(0.04)	0.04(0.06)	0.09(0.05)	0.03(0.07)
5	0.14(0.03)	0.05(0.05)	0.13(0.05)	0.03(0.06)	0.09(0.06)	0.05(0.08)
	Developmental Change					
Modes	Thickness		Surface Area		Volume	
	Train	Test	Train	Test	Train	Test
1	0.33(0.01)	0.29(0.03)	0.52(0.07)	0.48(0.09)	0.53(0.01)	0.51(0.04)
2	0.23(0.11)	0.14(0.14)	0.17(0.06)	0.05(0.08)	0.15(0.03)	0.04(0.05)
3	0.19(0.11)	0.07(0.15)	0.16(0.06)	0.05(0.09)	0.16(0.03)	0.05(0.05)
4	0.14(0.06)	0(0.09)	0.16(0.06)	0.05(0.09)	0.15(0.04)	0.04(0.06)
5	0.14(0.04)	-0.01(0.06)	0.15(0.05)	0.03(0.07)	0.15(0.04)	0.03(0.06)

4.6 Study 3 Acknowledgements, Disclosures and Funding

The full acknowledgements, disclosures and funding can be accessed via doi:

10.1038/s41380-020-0757-x

Chapter 5: Multivariate Patterns of Brain-Behavior-Environment Associations in the Adolescent Brain and Cognitive Development Study

<u>Originally published as:</u>

Amirhossein Modabbernia, Delfina Janiri, Gaelle E Doucet, Abraham Reichenberg, Sophia Frangou. Biol Psychiatry. 2021 Mar 1;89(5):510-520. doi: 10.1016/j.biopsych.2020.08.014. Epub 2020 Aug 24.

5.1 Study 4 Introduction

Adolescence is a period of significant brain reorganization that can be assessed using a range of neuroimaging measures [145,196-202]. Morphometric changes involve increase in brain volume, expansion of the cortical surface area and reduction in cortical thickness [145,196]. Maturational changes in intra-cortical myelination can be captured using the gray/white matter contrast while metrics derived from diffusion MRI inform about similar changes in white matter (WM) microstructure [202]. Intracortical myelination shows a prolonged developmental trajectory, primarily within prefrontal and other association regions, that facilitates the dynamic, experience dependent configuration of cognitive systems [197,200,201]. Developmental increases in the diameter and myelination of axons and in the fiber packing density of WM tracts are reflected in reductions in axial (AD) and radial (RD) water diffusivity and increases in fractional anisotropy (FA) [203]. Functional brain changes, primarily involve increased connectivity of the cognitive brain networks linked to improvements in the adaptive control of cognition and behavior [199].

Brain organization throughout the lifespan has been associated with multiple genetic, molecular, behavioral and environmental factors (9-18). Large-scale studies in adults have begun to address the complexity of the brain-behavior-environment associations. In the Human Connectome Project (www.humanconnectomeproject.org), a US study of over one thousand healthy adults aged 22-37 years, positive personal attributes and environmental factors were positively correlated with each other and with brain structure and connectivity; the reverse was observed for negative factors [159-161]. A study on the first 5,000 participants of the UK biobank (www.ukbiobank.ac.uk), a population-based study involving adults aged 40-69 years, reported multiple distinct modes of population covariation that reflected associations between multimodal measures of brain organization and life factors including physical characteristics, socioeconomic and cognitive variables [204].

Understanding the role of positive and negative life factors in shaping brain organization in early adolescence is particularly relevant to mental health as the origins of most mental disorders can be traced to this period [143]. Neuroscience-based public health policies to improve mental health outcomes critically depend on evidence from large-scale datasets. The Adolescent Brain and Cognitive Development (ABCD) Study (https://abcdstudy.org/) [205] is such a large dataset which provides high-quality neuroimaging data and detailed environmental and behavioral information from a nationally representative population-based sample of 9–10-year-olds (n=11,875) living in the USA. This rich dataset allowed us to test (a) whether patterns of covariation between a wide array of brain metrics with a broad range of personal characteristics and environmental exposures are robust and reproducible; (b) whether specific exposures show particularly strong and/or wide-ranging associations with adolescent brain organization; (c) whether covariation between exposures and brain metrics is spatially diffuse or shows evidence of regional specificity. To achieve this, we used multivariate analyses to identify patterns of covariation between multimodal neuroimaging metrics and a comprehensive array of non-imaging measures pertaining to perinatal and developmental history, physical and mental wellbeing, cognitive ability, parental characteristics, family functioning, neighborhood environment, and socioeconomic circumstances.

5.2 Study 4 Methods

5.2.1 Sample

The ABCD study recruited a nationally representative cohort of 11,875 youth aged 9-10 years at 22 US sites using multi-stage probability sampling (Supplemental Methods, Section 1). The analyses presented here, used data preprocessed by the ABCD downloaded in July 19 as part of the ABCD Study Curated Annual Release 2.0.1

(https://data-archive.nimh.nih.gov/abcd). We selected ABCD participants based on the availability of non-imaging measures and of high-quality neuroimaging data (Supplemental Methods, Section 4).

5.2.2 Non-Imaging Measures

We examined a total of 72 non-imaging measures (NIMs) pertaining to perinatal events (i.e., parental age at child's birth, planned pregnancy, maternal medical conditions during pregnancy, maternal use of prescribed medication, alcohol and substance use during pregnancy, premature birth, twin birth, caesarian delivery, obstetric complications, and birthweight), early development (duration of breastfeeding, motor and verbal development), anthropometric measures (i.e., pubertal stage, height, weight, waist circumference), psychopathology (i.e., eight subscales of the Child Behavior Checklist, and prodromal symptoms, subsyndromal mania, and sleep problems), cognition (i.e., fluid and crystallized cognition), psychological traits (i.e., negative urgency, lack of planning, lack of perseverance, sensation seeking, behavioral Inhibition, drive, reward responsiveness, positive affect, and prosocial behavior), common childhood medical conditions, school engagement and environment, life events, lifestyle (i.e., screen time on digital devices, number of friends, and physical activity), parental characteristics (i.e., education, and psychopathology, martial and educational status), family environment (i.e., finances, family conflict, and quality of parental engagement) and neighborhood environment (i.e., area deprivation, risk of lead exposure, pollution, safety, and crime) [206-208]. Detailed definition of the measures and the corresponding

assessment instruments are provided in Supplemental Methods and Supplemental

Tables S1.

5.2.3 Neuroimaging Measures

The availability of high-quality neuroimaging data differed for each modality

(Table 1). To maximize sample size, we analyzed each modality separately using

morphometric data from 9623 participants, gray/white matter contrast measures from

9215 participants, diffusion MRI measures from 7637 participants and resting-state

network (RSN) connectivity measures from 5742 participants. Structural (T_1w and T_2w),

diffusion (dMRI), and resting-state functional MRI data were collected, processed and

analyzed according to previously published and standardized ABCD protocols[20,24]

(details in Supplemental Methods, Section 4). Definitions of all the neuroimaging

measures are provided in Supplemental Table S2-S5.

Table 5.1. Demographic characteristics of each sample

	sMRI N=9623	Gray/White Matter Contrast N=9215	DWI N=7637	rs-fMRI N=5742
Age, Months, Mean (SD)	119 (7.5)	119 (7.5)	119 (7.5)	120 (7.5)
Sex, Female, N (%)	4766 (49%)	4542 (49%)	3836 (49%)	2981 (52%)
Race, White, N (%)	5043 (52%)	4872 (53%)	4258 (55%)	3173 (55%)
Race, Hispanic, N (%)	1402 (15%)	1339 (15%)	1013 (13%)	723 (13%)
Race, Black, N (%)	1991 (21%)	1883 (20%)	1587 (20%)	1145 (20%)
Race, Other, N (%)	1187 (12%)	1121 (12%)	911 (12%)	701 (12%)

sMRI=Structural Magnetic Resonance Imaging; DWI=Diffusion Weighted Imaging; rs-fMRI=resting state functional connectivity; Samples were selected after applying imaging quality exclusion criteria for each imaging modality separately (details in Supplementary Methods).

5.2.4 Statistical Analyses

A detailed step by step description of the statistical analyses is presented in Supplemental Methods (Section 5). Using an identical pipeline (Supplemental Figure S1), we conducted multivariate analyses between the NIMs and neuroimaging measures from each modality separately (i.e., brain morphometry derived from T1w images, myelination as inferred from gray/white contrast in T1-images, WM integrity derived from dMRI and RCN connectivity) (Supplemental Methods, Section 5.1). The code for the analysis is provided in the supplementary material. Briefly, each pipeline consisted of the following steps (a) division of the original datasets into a training (85% of the original) and a test (15% of the original) subsample; (b) missing value imputation using *bagImpute* in the Caret package (Version 6.0-84); (c) residualization for potential confounders; these comprised age, age^2, sex, age x sex, age^2 x sex, ethnicity, handedness, and scanner site for both imaging and non-imaging measures, and head motion and scanner type for the imaging data; (d) Principal Component Analysis (PCA) of the residualized values was implemented using the pca function from the mixOmics package (version 6.8.0); (e) Canonical Correlation Analysis (CCA) on the resulting principal components implemented using the CCA package (version 1.2) in R; (f) calculation of canonical structural loadings, i.e., the correlation coefficient between each variate and its corresponding variables, to quantify the contribution of each variable to each mode; (g) calculation of P-values for the CCA models was based on 10000 randomly permuted datasets (Supplemental Methods, Section 5.5); (h) Testing the generalizability of the CCA modes generated from the training subsample to the test subsample. The threshold for statistical significance, following False Discovery Rate (FDR)[209] correction for multiple testing, was set at $P_{FDR}<0.05$. Significant modes that explained at least 1% of the covariance were reported.

To ensure reliability and reproducibility, in addition to permutation testing mentioned above, we undertook further analyses described in detail in Supplemental Methods (Section 5.6). These included testing the stability of the PCA-CCA results (a) to sample composition using bootstrapping with replacement and random resampling; (b) to site using the leave-one out method; (c) to imputation by repeating the analyses using only non-imputed data; and (d) to family relatedness.

5.3 Study 4 Results

5.3.1 Brain Morphometry

We considered data from 9623 ABCD participants with high-quality global and regional measures of cortical thickness and surface area and subcortical volumes (Supplemental Figure S2, Supplemental Tables S2 and S6). Five modes, labelled morphometry modes (MM) 1 to 5, were statistically significant at $P_{FDR}<0.0001$ and replicable in the discovery (n=8144; $r_{discovery}$=0.26 to 0.46) and test sub-samples (n=1479; r_{test}=0.11 to 0.39) (Figure 1, Supplemental Figures S3-S5). In MM1, which explained the largest amount of covariance, the covariation pattern of the NIMs appeared aligned with traditional views of positive and negative life factors (Figure 1b). Specifically, the highest positive loadings comprised measures reflecting better cognition, better physical development (e.g., birthweight, height and weight) and enriched social environment (e.g., higher family income and parental education, planned pregnancy, greater parental warmth and engagement). Negative life factors with the highest loading comprised indices of personal (e.g., birth complications, higher psychopathology) and social disadvantage (e.g., neighborhood deprivation and family conflict). The direction of the morphometric loadings in MM1 were consistent with the expected development changes [145,196]; volumetric and cortical surface area measures showed positive loadings and cortical thickness measures showed negative loadings (Figure 1c). The largest negative loadings were observed for the cortical thickness of the cingulate, and of the medial, lateral and ventral prefrontal regions; the largest positive loadings were noted for total brain volume and global surface area. Of the remaining modes, MM5 mainly reflected associations with psychopathology and behavioral traits. The remaining modes (MM2, MM3 and MM4), explained residual variance relating to (a) positive covariation between cortical thickness and measures of cardiometabolic fitness (e.g., lower weight and waist circumference) in addition to better socioeconomic status, better cognition, and lower psychopathology in MM2 (Figure 1, Supplemental Figures S3-S5); (b) positive covariation of twin birth and high socioeconomic status and global morphometric measures in MM3 (Figure 1,

Supplemental Figures S3-S5); and (c) negative covariation between sub-syndromal mood

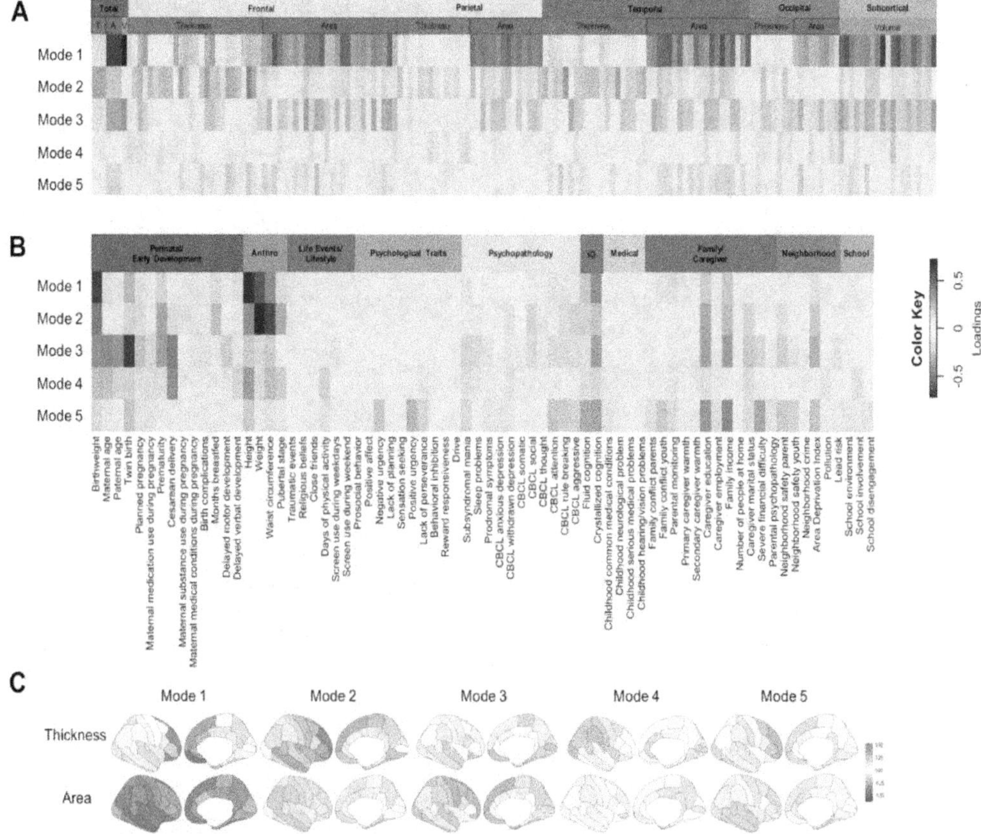

Figure 5.1. Significant Morphometry Modes.
a. Variable loadings for morphometry measures for the five significant morphometry modes (A,T,V refer to cortical surface area, cortical thickness, and subcortical volumes respectively). b. Variable loadings for non-imaging measures for the five significant morphometry modes; c. Loadings of the morphometry measures on regional cortical thickness and cortical surface area for the five significant modes. For the simplicity only the right hemisphere is shown. For a more detailed presentation see Supplemental Figures S4 and S5. CBCL: Childhood Behavior Checklist

symptoms, higher cognitive and school engagement and higher socioeconomic status

with cortical thickness in MM4 (Figure 1, Supplemental Figures S3-S5).

5.3.2 Gray/White Matter Contrast

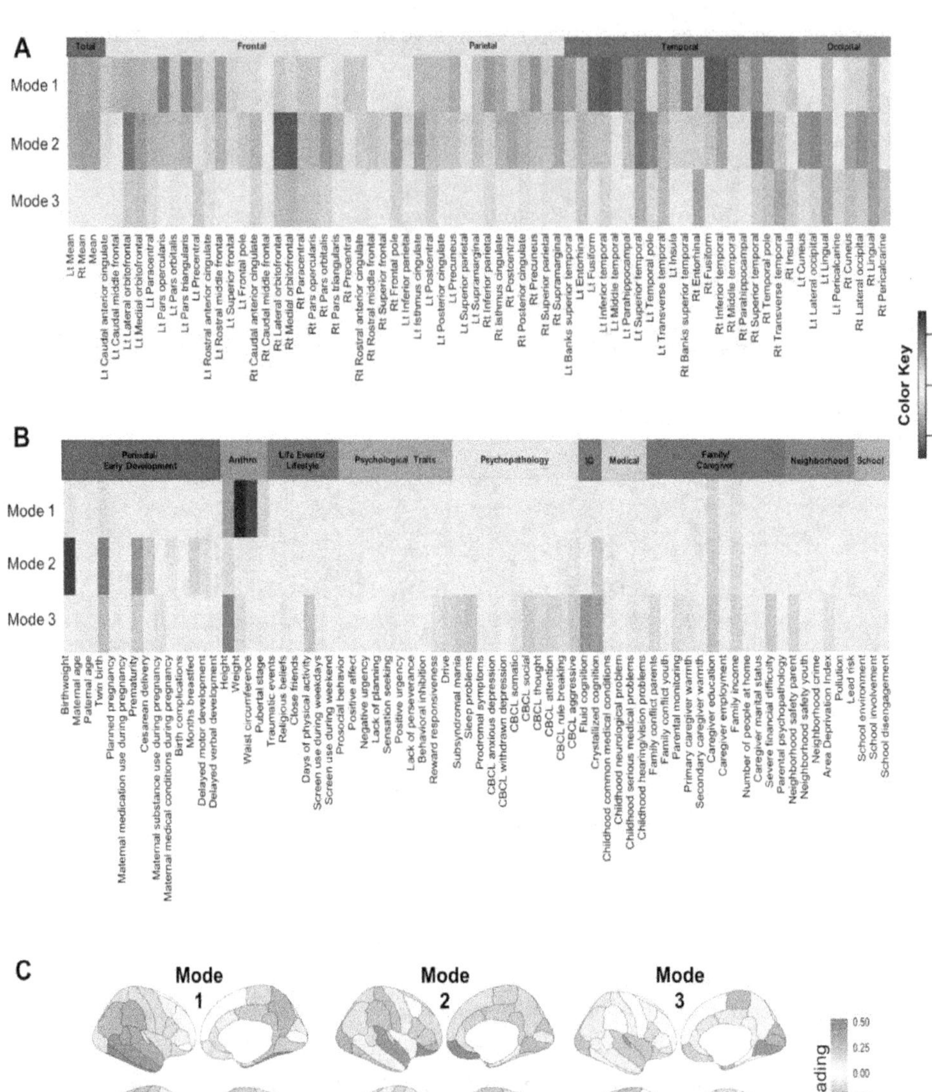

Figure 5.2. Significant Gray/White Matter Contrast Modes.

a. Variable loadings for gray/white matter contrast measures for the three significant gray/white matter contrast modes. b. Variable loadings for non-imaging measures for the three significant gray/white matter contrast modes; c. Loadings of the gray/white matter contrast measures depicted on the brain for the three significant modes. For a more detailed presentation see Supplemental Figures S6 and S7. CBCL: Childhood Behavior Checklist

We considered data from 9215 ABCD participants (Supplemental Figure S2,

Supplemental Tables S3 and S7) with high-quality gray/white matter contrast measures.

Three modes, labelled contrast mode (CM) 1 to 3, were statistically significant at

P_{FDR}<0.0001 in the discovery sub-sample (n= 7795; $r_{discovery}$ =0.21 to 0.37) and replicable in

the test (n=1420; r_{test} =0.10 to 0.20) sub-sample (Figure 2, Supplemental Figures S6-S7).

CM1 was dominated by negative loadings involving weight, height and waist

circumference and positive loadings on gray/white matter contrast measures of multiple

regions throughout the brain (Figure 2, Supplemental Figure S7). In CM2, higher positive

loadings in the gray/white matter contrast in orbitofrontal regions were most evident and

associated with positive loadings for birth weight and negative loadings for obstetric

events (prematurity and twin birth) (Figure 2, Supplemental Figure S7). CM3 captured

the association between height, better cognition, lower psychopathology, and higher

physical activity; gray/white matter contrast measures showed positive loadings in

orbitofrontal and entorhinal regions and negative loadings in the visual and transverse

temporal regions (Figure 2, Supplemental Figure S7).

5.3.3 White Matter Integrity

We considered data from 7637 ABCD participants (Supplemental Figure S2,

Supplemental Tables S4 and S8) with high quality dMRI measures. Four modes, labelled

WM modes (WMM) 1 to 4, were statistically significant at P_{FDR}<0.0001 and replicable in

in the discovery (n=6480; $r_{discovery}$=0.25 to 0.44) and test sub-samples (n= 1157; r_{test}=0.13 to

0.34) (Figure 3, Supplemental Figures S8-S9). In WMM1, the highest NIM loadings were negative and involved anthropometric measures (most prominently weight, waist circumference, height and pubertal stage); the highest positive loadings involved the AD of the corpus callosum and of the major WM tract fibers (Figure 3, Supplemental Figures S8-S9). In WMM2, NIMs representing positive perinatal factors (higher birthweight, longer duration of breastfeeding), better cognition and enriched social environment (family income and parental education and involvement) covaried with one another; similar covariation was observed amongst negative early life events (maternal medical problems and substance use, birth complications, and delayed development), psychopathology (particularly social, prodromal, attention and externalizing symptoms) and social disadvantage (greater area deprivation and severe financial difficulties). In WMM2, the highest positive and negative loadings respectively involved the FA and RD of large WM tracts, particularly those connecting prefrontal to other brain regions (Figure 3, Supplemental Figures S8-S9). WMM3 accounted for further variance attributable to perinatal events (with positive loadings for twin birth, prematurity and negative loading for birthweight) and their association with positive AD and FA but negative RD loadings for corticostriatal and corticospinal tracts (Figure 3, Supplemental Figures S8-S9). In WMM4, NIMs showed a positive-negative covariation pattern similar to WMM2, but with opposite signs on height, and FA in large white matter tracts (particularly the uncinate and cingulate bundles) (Figure 3, Supplemental Figures S8-S9).

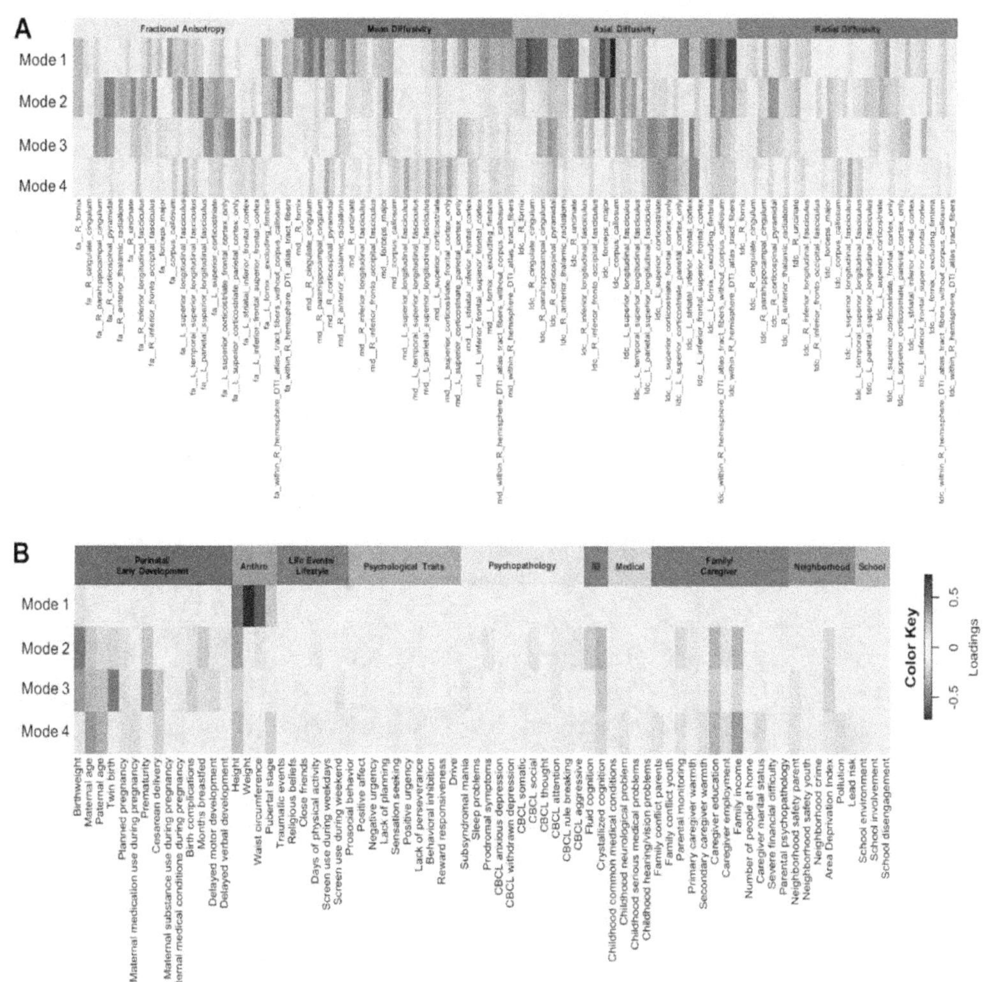

Figure 5.3. Significant White Matter Integrity Modes.
a. Variable loadings for white matter integrity measures for the four significant white matter integrity modes. b. Variable loadings for non-imaging measures for the four significant white matter integrity modes; For a more detailed presentation see Supplemental Figures S8 and S9. CBCL: Childhood Behavior Checklist

5.3.4 Resting-State Network Connectivity

We considered data from 5742 ABCD participants (Supplemental Figure S2, Supplemental Tables S5 and S9) with high-quality RSN connectivity measures. Two

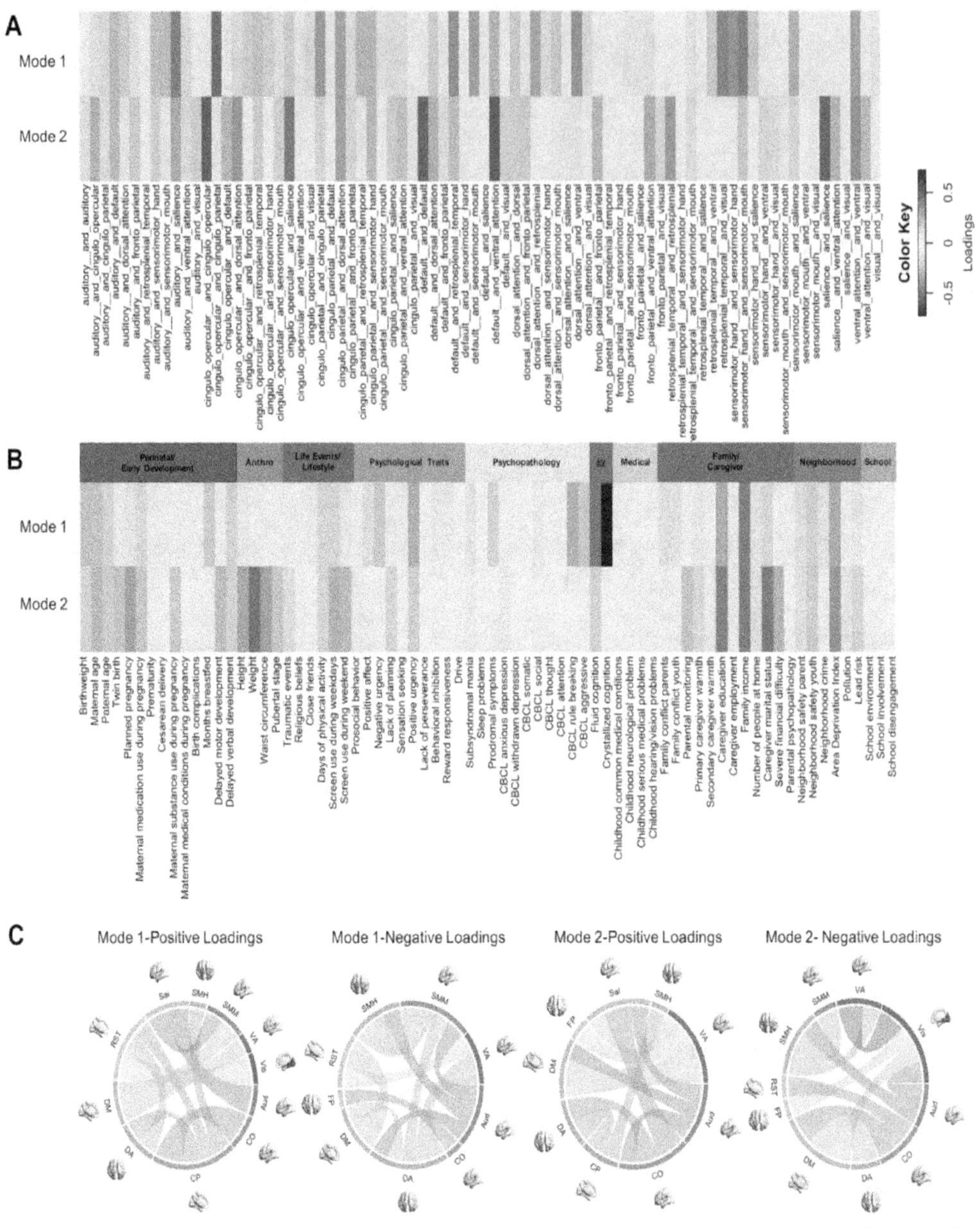

Figure 5.4. Significant Resting State Functional Connectivity Modes.
a. Variable loadings for resting state functional connectivity measures for the two significant for resting state functional connectivity modes; b. Variable loadings for non-imaging measures for the two significant resting state functional connectivity modes; c. Top ten between-network connectivity loadings for the two significant resting state functional connectivity modes. For a more detailed presentation see Supplemental Figures S10 and S11. CBCL: Childhood Behavior Checklist

The results reported above were robust to sample composition, imputation, site and relatedness as shown in Supplemental Figures S12-S15 and Supplementary Tables S10-S11.

5.4 Study 4 Discussion

Multivariate data-driven analyses identified 14 patterns of brain-behavior-environment covariation in a large US population-based cohort of young adolescents. The findings were robust to sample size and composition and independent of site. In line with studies in adults [159,160], the patterns identified indicate that regardless of neuroimaging modality, life factors typically considered positive were associated with brain measures that reflect advantageous brain development while the reverse was the case for factors considered negative.

A particular strength of the study is that the rich ABCD dataset enabled us to expand prior literature that focused on associations between limited sets of imaging measures and non-imaging variables. By quantifying the associations between multiple brain measures with a wide range of NIMs in an integrated analysis framework, we demonstrated that neither positive nor negative exposures occur in isolation. Positive exposures tended to covary with one another and the same was the case for negative exposures (Figures 1b-4b). Although their relative contribution varied across modes, the direction of association was usually consistent with their hypothesized effects; positive exposures were positively associated with measures reflecting favorable brain development while the reverse was the case for negative exposures. Of note, both positive and negative factors showed spatially diffuse patterns of covariation with brain measures. We were able to demonstrate this by retaining global measures of brain thickness and volume in our models as opposed to removing their variance by residualizing regional measures. Together, these observations suggest that attributions of specificity in correlations between single NIMs and brain measures may need to be revisited and future studies would benefit from focusing on the wider context in which brain development occurs.

Factors most consistently associated with neuroimaging measures across modalities involved socioeconomic circumstances, the quality of parental engagement, perinatal events, cognitive ability and psychopathology. In modes where psychopathology loadings were present, they typically covaried with lower cognition and lower quality of family and neighborhood environments. We suggest that these commonly co-occurring exposures, and their effect on the brain, should be considered in models of brain-psychopathology. Within modes, the different measures of psychopathology also covaried with one another, in line with arguments for a common latent dimension for psychopathology [210]. The association between general psychopathology and lower cognitive abilities has been documented in other population-based cohorts, notably the Dunedin Multidisciplinary Health and Development Study [211].

However, two modes went against this general pattern. In MM4, we observed covariation of affective and sleep problems, better academic ability, higher socioeconomic status and greater cortical thinning. These findings resonate with epidemiological evidence linking higher cognitive and academic performance in adolescence with the emergence of bipolar morbidity in adulthood [212,213]. MM5 captured the remaining covariance relating to dysregulation in attention and impulse control, and social adversity. This pattern has also been identified in epidemiological studies in connection to childhood disorders such as ADHD and disruptive mood dysregulation disorder [214], and mood and substance use disorders in adulthood [215].

We confirmed the known links between higher cognitive ability and brain development across modalities [38,155]. Although we highlight here the associations of cognitive ability with RSN connectivity and gray/white matter contrast because of their high loadings in FM1 and CM3 modes, we emphasize that these occurred within the context of advantageous socioeconomic and family conditions. In FM1, better cognitive ability was associated with increased connectivity between networks that support higher-order cognitive functions associated with salience processing (cingulo-opercular and salience networks) and executive control (cingulo-parietal network). The higher integration of these networks is consistent with their evolving role in coordinating multiple mental operations in the maturing brain [199]. In CM3, higher gray/white matter contrast intensity in prefrontal regions was also associated with better cognition. Higher gray/white matter contrast intensity is thought to represent lower levels of intracortical myelin [216,217]. The lower myelin concentration in the prefrontal cortices, together with their prolonged maturation pattern, is thought to facilitate flexible, experience-dependent configuration of prefrontally-linked cognitive systems [201,218].

Anthropometric measures made major contributions to multiple modes across modalities confirming body-brain associations during development [219]. We did not remove the variance of these variables from the sample as it was important to demonstrate the strength of their associations with brain organization which is greater than that of many other factors. This perspective is important when making inferences about the strength of the associations of different factors with brain measures which often tend to over-emphasize factors of much smaller magnitude. We highlight the loadings of weight and waist circumference on morphometry (MM2, MM3), axial diffusivity (WMM1) and intra-cortical myelin (CM1). These measures, which are considered indices of "cardiometabolic fitness" [220], appear to influence brain organization even at the early stages of adolescence.   We also note the persistent association between brain morphometry (MM1 and MM2) and white matter integrity (WMM2) with perinatal events, and particularly prematurity, birthweight and twin births. These findings add to the substantial body of evidence linking perinatal events to health outcomes throughout the lifespan [221,222].

It is important to consider key study limitations that point to avenues for future research. Covariation is not evidence of causation although we assume that many of the reported associations are underpinned by biological, and likely causative, mechanisms. The modes identified here are based on cross-sectional data; however, as the ABCD study has a longitudinal design, it would be possible to track the evolution of brain-behavior-environment covariation when follow-up data become available. Conversely, brain development is influenced by multiple factors that have been in operation prior to the enrollment age of the ABCD participants. It is conceivable that some of the results reported here are conditional on or influenced by very early exposures which are not fully captured here. We did not model specific domains of cognition that may characterize individual cognitive profiles more precisely [223]. Nevertheless, global measures of cognition show significant covariation with domain-specific measures which supports the usefulness of global measures in informing public health strategies. The macro-scale measures examined here are widely used in development neuroscience but do not capture brain-behavior-environment associations that may operate at a micro-structural level. Prior research on brain-behavior-environment associations has been criticized for over-estimating their effect size and for paying insufficient attention to their reproducibility [224,225]. In response, we undertook extensive reliability resting and we report those canonical modes that were reliable and generalizable. We ensured the stability and the reproducibility of the analyses using multiple techniques including permutation, resampling stability and replicability testing by splitting the sample into independent subsets. It is conceivable that our analyses may have missed certain brain-behavior-environment associations that may only exist within distinct but small and yet unknown subpopulations.

In summary, because of the richness of the imaging and non-imaging data available in the ABCD study and the large size of the cohort we were able to examine brain-behavior-environment association in youth in greater depth than has been previously possible. We identified 14 modes that represent patterns of covariation between different aspects of brain organization and behavioral and environmental factors. We show that most these factors tend to occur along patterns of increased advantage or adversity. Modeling life factors in isolation is therefore likely to miss the importance on the wider context in which they occur. Exposures relating to neighborhood environment, parental characteristics, quality of family life, perinatal history, cardiometabolic health, cognition and psychopathology had the most consistent association with brain organization and could be considered as priority targets for universal interventions to improve mental wellbeing in youth.

5.5 Study 4 Supplemental Material

Due to very large volume of the supplemental files, important tables and figures

are presented below and the rest are available only online. The full supplemental material

for this study can be accessed online through the following links: https://ars.els-

cdn.com/content/image/1-s2.0-S0006322320318461-mmc1.pdf

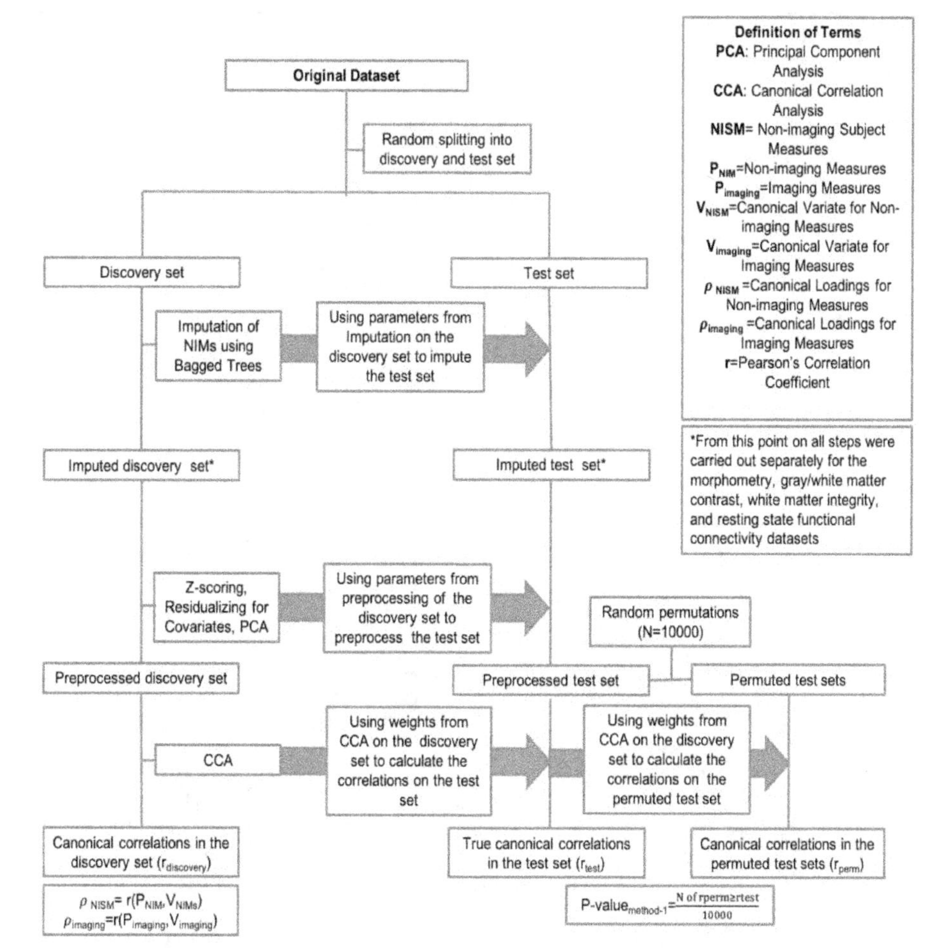

$$\rho_{NISM}= r(P_{NIM}, V_{NIMs})$$
$$\rho_{imaging}=r(P_{imaging}, V_{imaging})$$

$$P\text{-value}_{method-1}=\frac{N\ of\ rperm \geq rtest}{10000}$$

Figure S1A. Analysis Pipeline And Permutation Testing Method 1: See Supplemental Methods for details

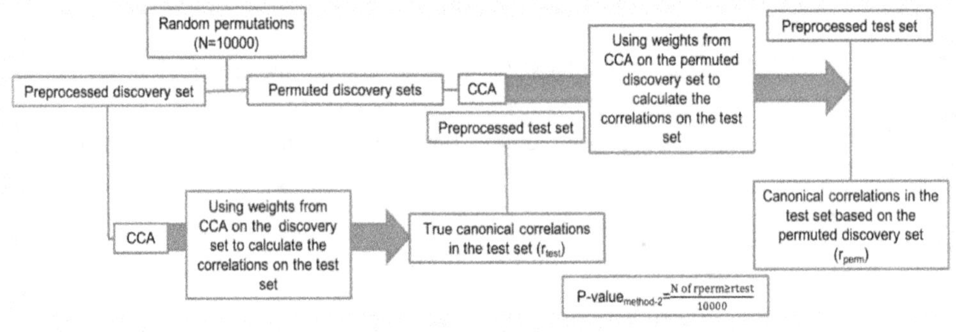

Figure S1B. Permutation Testing Method 2: See Supplemental Methods for details

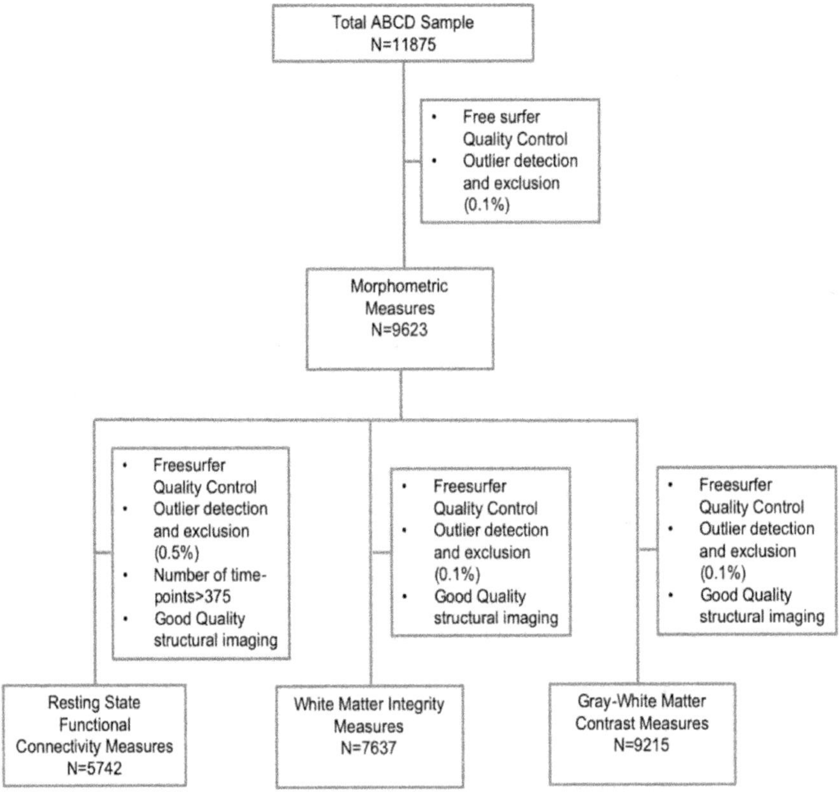

Figure S2. Flowchart of Sample Selection (details in Supplemental Methods, Selection of Study Samples)

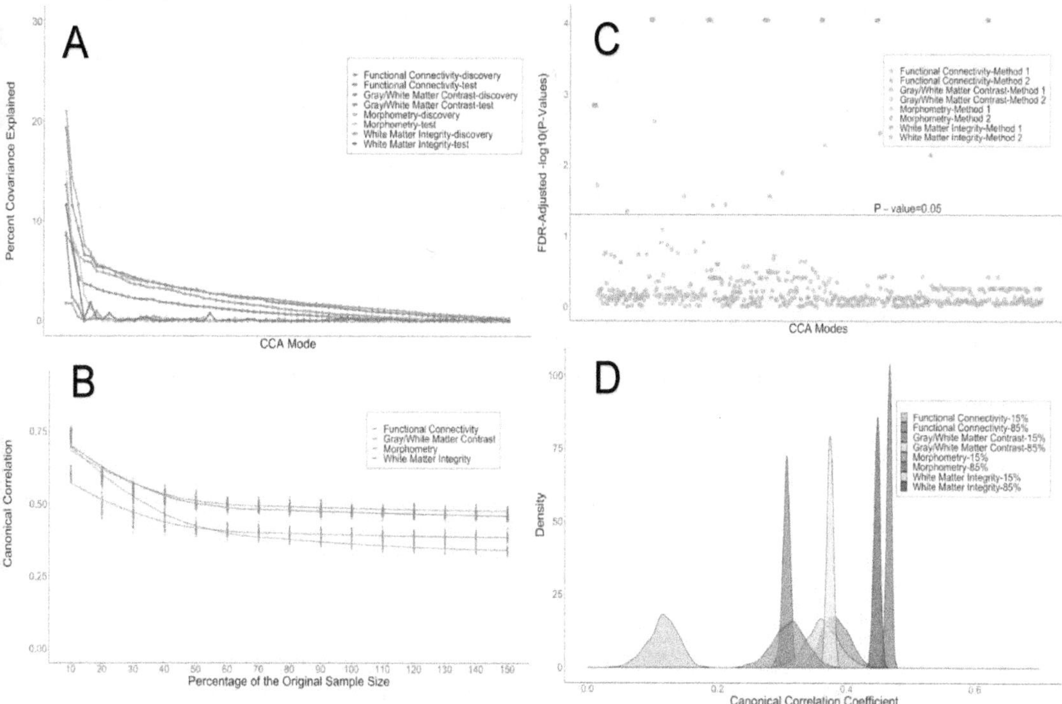

Figure S12. Ancillary analyses. A. Covariance explained by each mode in the discovery set and the test set; B. Canonical correlation on each modality as a function of sample size using a bootstrapping approach (sampling with replacement); C. P-values calculated using feature weights from the original model on the discovery set on the permuted the test set (Method 1) or using feature weights from the permuted discovery set on the unpermuted test set (Method 2); D. Canonical correlations for the first mode in 1000 randomly sampled discovery and test sets.

Table S10. Permutation-based calculation of p-values for the first ten modes in the test sets: False Discovery Rate Corrected P-values were calculated using feature weights from the model from the discovery set on the permuted the test set (Method 1) or using feature weights from the permuted discovery set on the unpermuted test set (Method 2). More details are provided in section 5.5 Assessing Statistical Significance Using Random Permutation Testing

Mode	Morphometry Method 1	Morphometry Method 2	Gray/White Matter Contrast Method 1	Gray/White Matter Contrast Method 2	White Matter Integrity Method 1	White Matter Integrity Method 2	Resting State Functional Connectivity Method 1	Resting State Functional Connectivity Method 2
1	0	0.00144	0	0	0	0	0	0.0072
2	0	0.00144	0	0	0	0	0	0.0072
3	0	0.00144	0	0	0	0	0.3744	0.495
4	0	0.00144	0.7525	0.783079	0.394667	0.3924	0.769846	0.812229
5	0	0.00144	0.3731	0.452375	0	0	0.54144	0.548182
6	0.0024	0.0192	0.0035	0.00525	0.312923	0.297818	0.54144	0.548182
7	0.675095	0.684857	0.538364	0.600727	0.323621	0.3924	0.54144	0.548182
8	0.589067	0.6384	0.3731	0.500889	0.0276	0.0372	0.54144	0.548182

Table S10. Permutation-based calculation of p-values for the first ten modes in the test sets: False Discovery Rate Corrected P-values were calculated using feature weights from the model from the discovery set on the permuted the test set (Method 1) or using feature weights from the permuted discovery set on the unpermuted test set (Method 2). More details are provided in section 5.5 Assessing Statistical Significance Using Random Permutation Testing

| 9 | 0.4448 | 0.588096 | 0.843962 | 0.886577 | 0.312923 | 0.386585 | 0.856653 | 0.814447 |
| 10 | 0.550656 | 0.588096 | 0.83566 | 0.805146 | 0.734965 | 0.788954 | 0.54144 | 0.548182 |

5.6 Study 4 Acknowledgements, Disclosures and Funding

The full acknowledgements, disclosures and funding can be accessed via doi:

10.1016/j.biopsych.2020.08.014

Chapter 6. Conclusions and Future Directions

The work comprising the Doctoral Thesis described herein contributes to a growing body of literature on how the brain changes during adolescence and how brain organization during this critical period relates to individual and their living environment.

In the first study, using brain structural data from more than 17,000 healthy subjects aged 3-90 years from the ENIGMA Lifespan working group, we mapped normative trajectories and reference curves for cortical thickness in 68 regions. We observed a general pattern wherein cortical thickness had its peak during childhood, and decreased with a steep slope during the first 2-3 decades of life and more gradually afterwards.

In the second study, we leveraged the resources of the ENIGMA Consortium to examine the age-related trajectories inferred from cross-sectional measures of subcortical structures from more than 18,000 individuals aged 3-90 years. Two major patterns were noticeable. The volume of the basal ganglia showed a monotonic negative association with age; there was no significant association between age and the volumes of the thalamus, amygdala and the hippocampus (with some degree of decline in thalamus) until the sixth decade of life followed by a steep negative association with age.

Future directions generated by the first two studies:

1. What is the biological mechanism underlying change in cortical and subcortical structures?

2. What does the deviation from the norm mean in terms of cognition, behavior, psychopathology, and functional outcomes?

3. How can we refine our models to make them more generalizable for potential use in clinical practice?

In the third study, we focused on adolescence as a critical period of vulnerability to psychopathology and significant brain reorganization. Specifically, we sought to discover linked patterns of covariation between brain structural development and a wide array of individual and environmental factors by leveraging data from the IMAGEN study, a longitudinal population-based cohort of adolescents. We observed that age, physical growth and sex had the highest association with changes in the adolescent brain structure; at baseline, further significant positive associations were noted for cognitive measures while negative associations were observed at both time points for prenatal parental smoking, life events, and negative affect and substance use.

Finally, we expanded on the findings of the third study by leveraging diverse measures of individual characteristics, environmental factors and brain structure and function in the ABCD sample, which is much larger than the IMAGEN sample. We observed that positive and negative exposures converged to form patterns of psychosocial advantage or adversity and that these exposures/behavioral patterns showed modality-general, respectively positive or negative, associations with brain structure and function with little evidence of regional specificity. We highlight the importance of understanding the complex and intertwined influences on brain organization and mental function during development which has the potential to inform public health policies aiming toward interventions to improve mental well-being. Future directions generated by the last two studies:

1. What factors contribute to more favorable/unfavorable brain developmental profiles in a given individual?

2. What is the role of genetics in brain-behavior-environment associations?

3. How can we leverage multimodal data encompassing biological and environmental information for prediction of mental health and functional outcomes in youth?